Fit For Life

Daley Thompson with
Sally Ann Voak

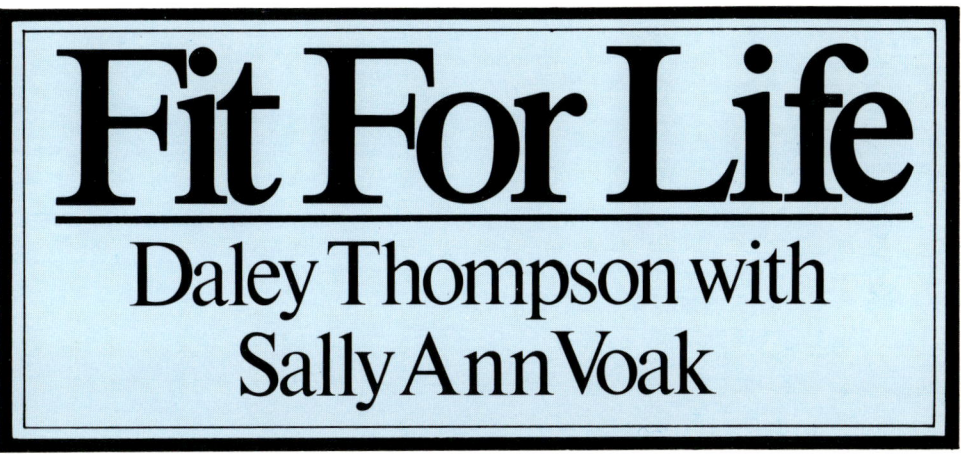

Fit For Life

Daley Thompson with Sally Ann Voak

Photography by Steve Powell, All-Sport

HODDER AND STOUGHTON

LONDON SYDNEY AUCKLAND TORONTO

Acknowledgements

Daley and Sally would like to thank:

Sylvia Caplin and Pineapple West, 60 Paddington Street, W1

The Hogarth Club, 1a Airedale Avenue, Chiswick, W4

Coulsdon Colts FC, Toldene, Old Coulsdon, Surrey

The Olympus Sport Shop at Selfridges, Oxford Street, London W1

The National Recreation Centre, Crystal Palace, London SE19

Biggin Hill School of Flying, Biggin Hill Airport, Surrey

And, most important, Snowy Brooks, Sheila Birkenshaw, Maureen Waller, Sharyn Troughton, Doreen Rayment, Patrick Ward-Lee, and Frank Dick

DESIGNER: BOB HOOK

ILLUSTRATOR: JANE TYRRELL

British Library Cataloguing in Publication Data

Thompson, Daley
  Fit for Life.
  1. Physical Fitness
  I. Title   II. Voak, Sally Ann
  613.7   RA781

  ISBN 0 340 34155 6

Contents

Foreword
by Jeffrey Archer

This is the only time in my life that I am going to be 'in front' of the greatest athlete in the world.

All those who care about the success of our national sportsmen cannot fail to respond to the achievements of Daley Thompson (I just wish he was not so good looking), and in our wildest fantasies would even like to emulate him.

This book will not win you a gold medal at the Los Angeles Olympics, because they are already stamping Daley's name on that, but what it will guarantee – if you are sensible enough to follow its sage advice – is a better opportunity for you to be fit for life.

With this book Daley Thompson could do for the men of Britain what Jane Fonda has done for the women of America.

Once you have read the book slowly and carefully, immediately return to 'Your Daley dozen'. If you stick to the routine as shown on pages 31 to 37, you will find that in a very short time you will have lost weight, your breathing will have improved and your muscles will look more like muscles and not just lumps of plasticine on a children's model of a grown-up.

One thing you must do when you have completed the book is tear out the 'Daley dozen' pages – for three reasons:

1 You can pin them on to the wall in your bedroom and not forget or avoid completing them each day.
2 Once those magic pages have been removed, no one will bother to pinch your copy.
3 And then Daley will sell more books.

I recommend *Fit For Life* to (a) anyone who sits down for more than one hour a day, (b) is more than four pounds overweight, (c) watches more hours of television than partakes in active exercise. That has taken care of ninety per cent of Britain, including YOU.

Even if we have to be armchair watchers at the next Olympics, Daley Thompson's *Fit For Life* will give us all the opportunity to be in much better shape for celebrating his next gold medal.

Jeffrey Archer ran the 100 yards for Somerset, Oxford and Great Britain in the early sixties, and is now President of Somerset AAA. In his spare time he writes novels.

Get fit for life with the world's fittest man

Sally Ann Voak writes:

He has been called the 'world's fittest man', 'superman', and he is undoubtedly the greatest all-round athlete the world has ever seen. Yet, Daley Thompson is the kind of athlete you do not feel foolish chatting to about your own, very humble, fitness problems. He is patient, fun, immensely knowledgeable, and has an instant rapport with children, teenagers and adults alike. Writing this book with him, I have been delighted (and a bit surprised) by his genuine concern for us 'ordinary' fairly unfit mortals and our attempts to get into shape; his advice is unfailingly practical, always takes into account the limited time at most people's disposal, and makes the quest for fitness a highly pleasurable process instead of a chore.

There is no one in the world better qualified than Daley to advise the whole family on keeping fit: the ten decathlon skills cover just about every kind of muscular movement and demand total co-ordination between body and mind (indeed, the whole purpose of the event is to test every aspect of man's athletic prowess). So, whether you need to brush up your running or soccer style, or want to tone up after having a baby, or just feel that you would like to get more out of life by improving your general fitness level, Daley has the answer.

He also has a way of putting over his ideas which is compulsively infectious: during the photographic sessions we all joined in the exercises, the swimming, the running, the soccer, the dance – whether we were in the pictures or not. It is just impossible to sit still in the presence of so much enthusiasm.

We hope the book gives *you* that kind of inspiration. Use it as a constant source of information wherever you happen to be. Make the most of your life – by becoming *Fit For Life*.

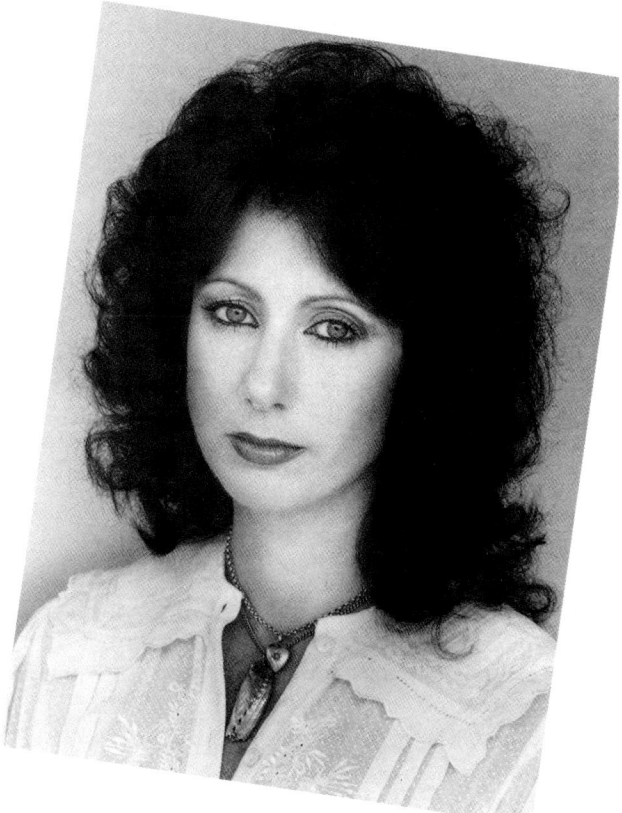

Daley Thompson writes:

I am a very lucky man. I actually spend most of my life enjoying something that most people can only manage in their spare time – sport. Admittedly, I have to work hard to try and improve my performance – it is impossible to describe the tiredness I feel after taking part in a big sports event – but the personal rewards more than make up for it.

My interest in sport in general was initially encouraged by my aunt, Mrs Doreen Rayment, who has looked after me for many years. She worked for the Kensington and Chelsea Play Association, which is a charitable trust to promote play facilities for children, and, inevitably, I was very much involved in these activities when I was a youngster. At that stage, I had no intention of becoming a decathlete. The training I did then was mostly orientated towards running, and a few weights. My very first coach was a chap called Pete Thompson from Worthing, and then Bob Mortimer of the Essex Beagles Athletics Club, who still helps me with my running and is a good friend. Like many teenagers, I became mad on football and actually had trials for Chelsea and Fulham, playing for Fulham juniors.

The idea of becoming a multi-event champion did not really enter my head until later. I could have been a good pole-vaulter, maybe a sprinter, and I do make the British team now as a specialist long-jumper – but, eventually, there was an irresistible attraction in knowing that I could, possibly, be the very best in the world at the decathlon.

If you have ever watched the decathlon, or seen it on television, you will know that it is a two-day event consisting of ten different skills. On day one, there are the 100 metre sprint, long jump, shot putt, high jump, and the 400 metres. On day two, there are the 110 metre hurdles, the discus, pole vault, javelin, and the 1,500 metres. Points are awarded according to tables worked out in 1962, based on the average of the world's top 100 people in each event. My big ambition (apart from winning the Gold at the 1984 Olympics) is to push my points up to a total of 9,000. The decathlon is never really afforded the kind of press and attention which I think it deserves, and that is why I am even more determined to win the Olympic

Gold next year in Los Angeles, and why I have to follow a very vigorous training programme of my own in preparation for the Games.

These days, I still live with Aunt Doreen in Surrey, but my training (nine hours a day, every day of the year) takes place in a variety of places, according to where the best facilities are: partly at the New River Sports Centre in Haringey, North London; partly in Crawley; and for three months of the year in California, with my buddy and shot putt and discus coach, Richard Slaney. Richard will be helping me again next year when I go to California in training for the Olympics in July.

In *Fit For Life*, I have tried to pass on just about everything I know about keeping fit. It is based on the experiences I have had, the skills I have learnt, and the knowledge I have acquired from talking to and working with some of the world's top sportsmen and sportswomen.

The full benefits of exercise are probably still underestimated, but I firmly believe that the fitter your body, the better chance you have of leading a long and healthy life. Exercise improves muscle tone, body shape and weight distribution, and there are also hidden benefits in it, such as release from stress, increased mental as well as physical energy, and greater resistance to disease. Although I have included a section on sensible eating in this book, one of the big plus factors about exercise is that, taken regularly, it can solve your weight problems once and for all.

You must be sensible about your aims in a fitness programme. If you are young and active, there is no reason why you should not be as fit as me (or almost), but do remember that I am at this peak of fitness for a specific purpose – it is unlikely that you will ever have to do anything which is quite so gruelling. Aim instead for a level which enables you to enjoy life, to run for a bus without being puffed out, to play a sport, and to rough and tumble with your children. If you are a child yourself, aim to be a good all-rounder – do not specialise in one particular field until you are older. If you are older, and lead a sedentary life, think about mobility. For instance, even if I lose fifty per cent of my present mobility by the time I am seventy, I shall still be very sprightly indeed and be able to enjoy life. You can look forward to being just as mobile in your old age if you work to reach your maximum fitness potential *now*.

Not all the advice in *Fit For Life* applies to everyone – select the exercise routines, the schedules, the dietary advice which are most suitable for you and your lifestyle. (Check with your doctor before tackling any of the exercises in this book if you have a history of back trouble.) Whatever programme you decide upon, stick to it. I would rather you aimed low – a few daily exercises, for instance (see Your Daley dozen on page 31) – than aimed too high and gave up the struggle after a few weeks. Look at the list of clubs and sports facilities on page 127, too, to widen your scope. Always think of exercise as a sociable activity; you will see that we are having fun in the photographs, and that is the way it should be. Never let exercise become a drudge, a routine to be endured; even an athlete like myself has to be careful to maintain a broad span of other interests, because I think you can become very bored, and boring, if you just stick to your 'job', even if that job happens to be a sport.

Keep *Fit For Life* around for the whole family to dip in to. It opens flat, so that you can follow

each exercise easily. Take the book on holiday, so that you can do some exercise when you have most time to spare, use it on a daily basis at home or at work, and when you want to put in extra training at school. *Fit For Life* is not just a practical work-book but a fun guide to healthy, happy living.

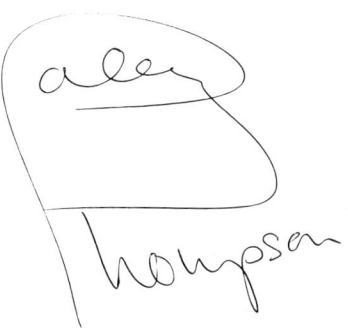

HIGHLIGHTS OF DALEY'S CAREER

1978   Wins Commonwealth Games title in Canada, at the age of 19, with a points total of 8,467.

1980   Wins the Olympic title in Moscow, points total 8,410.

1982   Wins title and sets a new World Record at the European Games in Athens, points total 8,744.

1982   Maintains title with points total of 8,410 at the Commonwealth Games in Australia.

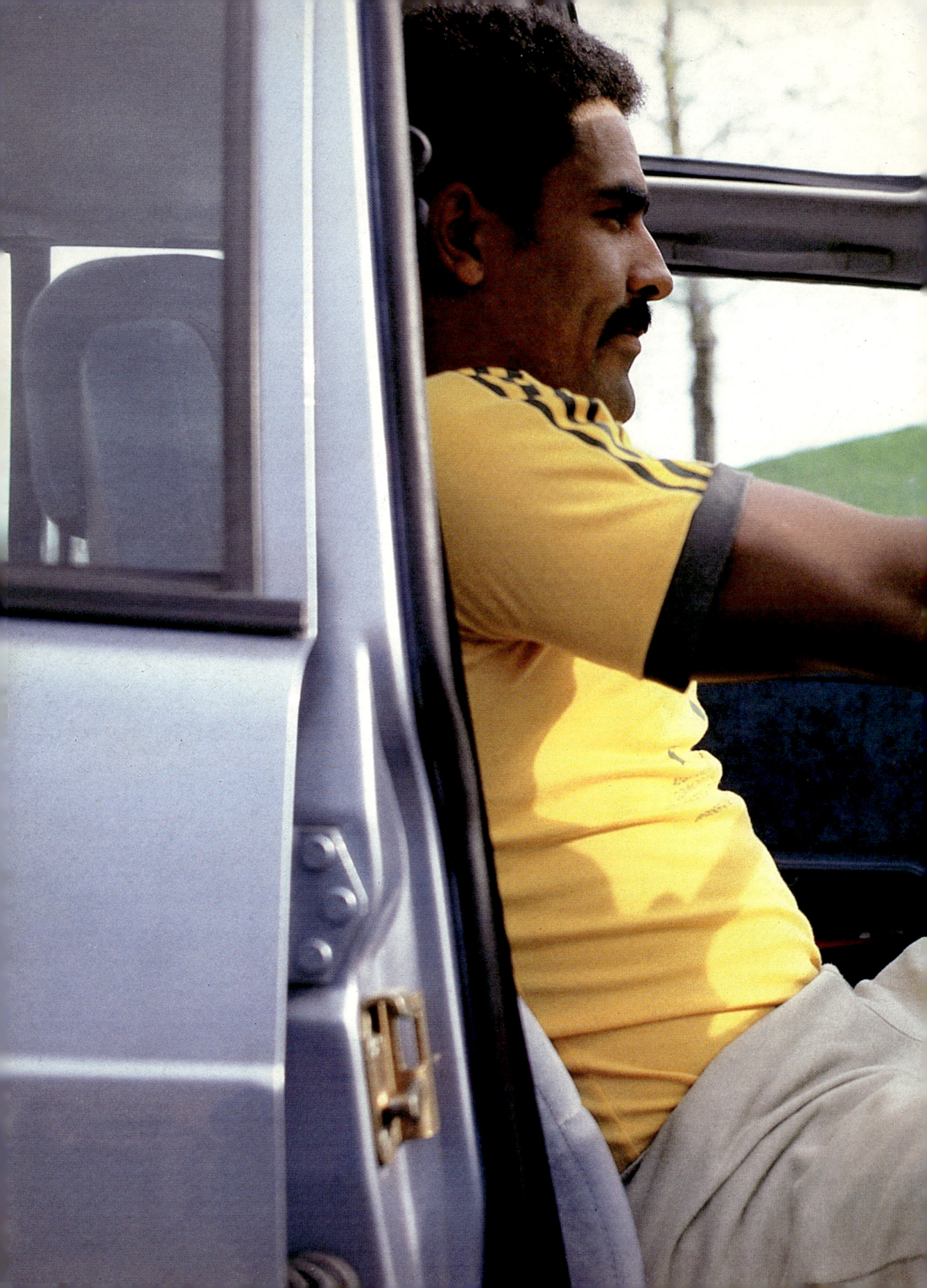

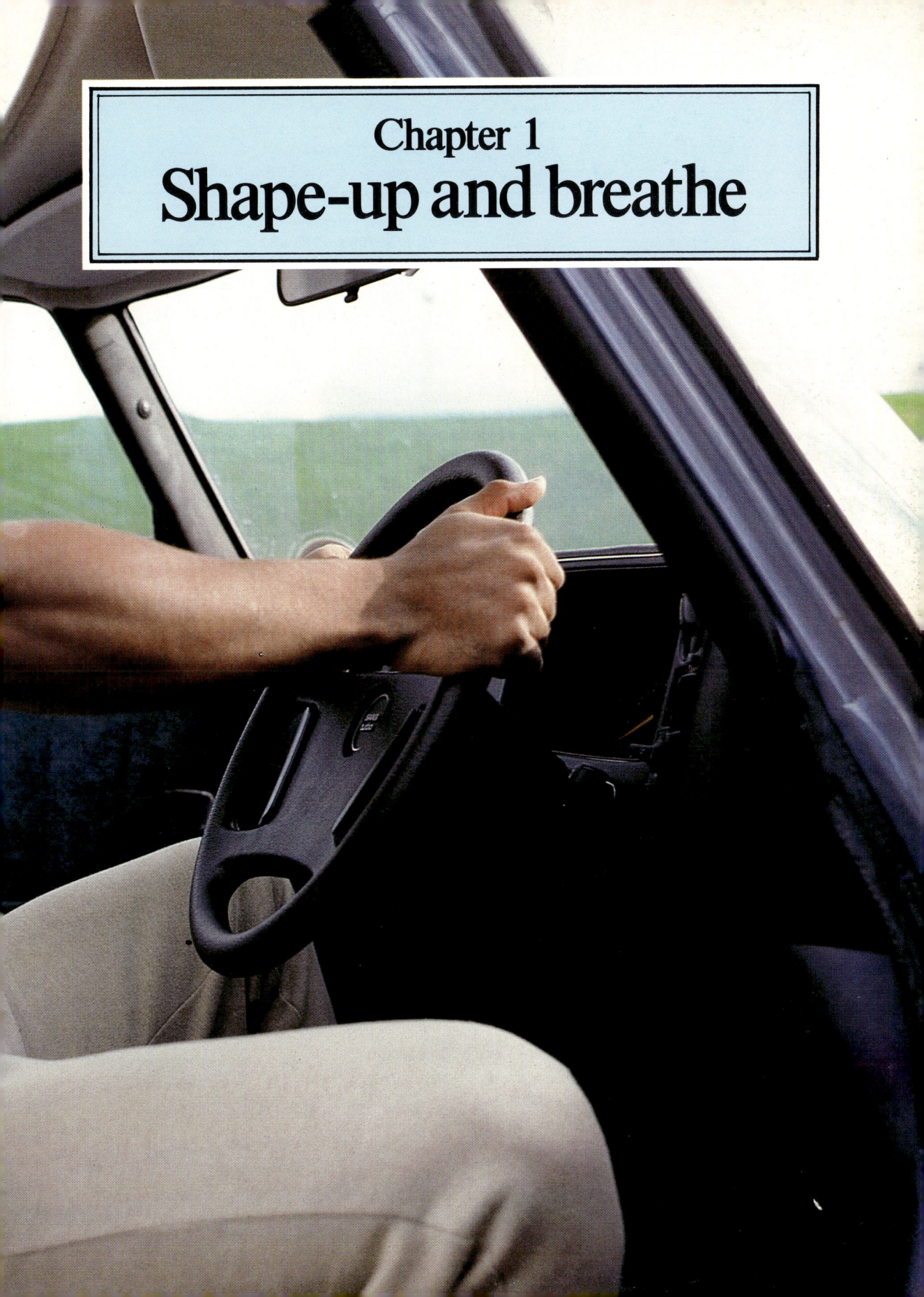

Chapter 1
Shape-up and breathe

The human body starts off in pretty good shape – babies are miracles of engineering perfection – but time and circumstances can alter it alarmingly, usually for the worse. Most people do not realise how much their posture, the way they move, and certain aspects of the environment can influence their body shape. Even before you consider taking exercise, you should know something about the machinery which actually controls your bodily movements, and how to make sure that it gets a fighting chance of working properly during your everyday life. Many of the problems which affect your health and enjoyment of life can be avoided if you learn to use your body well. Obviously, it is an advantage if this kind of body-knowledge starts at an early age when habits are formed, though in my experience children usually move well without being consciously aware of the fact – it is only later that they acquire bad posture, or start to develop awkward, harmful back movements. Luckily, it is never too late to improve bad habits, and many hours of back pain, in particular, can be avoided if you take the trouble to try.

POSTURE AND MOVEMENT

Although we take it for granted, the way we move is a complex process. The muscles do not contract until they receive a nerve message from the brain – and even the smallest movement needs action by at least two sets of muscles. Most require many more. For instance, just to walk one step, the following sequence takes place: first, that vital message is sent from the brain to the muscles of the feet, ankles, calves, thighs, hips, back, arms and neck – yes, they all take part. As you bring one leg upward and forward, the hip and knee joints of that leg must be bent and the weight of the body is tilted forward. For this to happen, muscle contraction must take place across the front of the groin and the back of the knee, muscle relaxation must occur across the back of the groin and the front of the knee. All the muscles of the feet and ankles must contract or relax, some of the arm, neck and trunk muscles relax, and others contract to bring the body forward so that you can keep your balance. Meanwhile, the muscles of the *other* leg are contracting or relaxing in readiness for the next step. Phew, the body has to do a lot of work just for that very simple movement!

If you are going to help your body move efficiently, you must first of all be sure that your

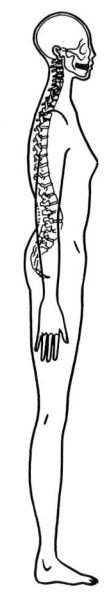

The human backbone is naturally curved in an 'S' shape. Do not stand ram-rod straight, but always relax your shoulders and keep your torso comfortably erect, hips steady, stomach tucked in.

posture is good. Ideally, your body should be stretched upwards so that the backbone is in its natural curves, but not held stiffly. Your weight should be evenly balanced on both feet, hip girdle held evenly, with both hips on the same level, the buttock muscles contracted slightly, stomach muscles held in, shoulders kept down and back a little (but not forced back), and arms held loosely by your sides. If an imaginary straight line was drawn from your ear to the ground, it would pass through your neck, shoulder joint, elbow, hand, hip joint, knee and the front of your ankle. Try this posture and see how much more comfortable it feels than a slouch. This is because your body is being kept upright by a very slight contraction of nearly all the body muscles and no one set of muscles is overworked. You will find you can stand like this for a couple of hours watching soccer or queuing for a seat for the Cup Final without feeling tired!

A good walking posture is the same, but the weight of your body should be tilted slightly forward as your weight is changed from the back to the front foot. Your arms should swing comfortably, but not exaggeratedly, and your toes must point forward. This is so important that I really cannot emphasise it enough. If you walk penguin-fashion (and most people do), or with your toes turned in, your whole body frame has to adjust to cope. What's more, the joints of your toes may become deformed, and corns develop. You may also form a layer of hard skin on your feet which can be painful, and your circulation will suffer, causing cold feet and chilblains. I am making a big point about this because healthy feet are vital to the enjoyment of nearly every sport I can think of. You can check your own foot movement style by looking at your shoes, as well as in the mirror: note how the soles and heels of your footwear are worn and make a definite attempt to correct any imbalance in future.

Other horrors of bad standing and walking posture include tiredness (if your shoulders sag forward your chest will be cramped, and lungs unable to expand fully – the body cells will not get enough oxygen, and you will feel less energetic); indigestion (if your backbone is not upright, your stomach and intestines will be cramped – food will not be churned up and moved along them properly, and you will get wind and stomach ache); and even arthritis (constant wobbling of the hip girdle may loosen the joints between the backbone and girdle leading to a lot of unnecessary pain later).

Another consequence of bad posture is that the body will often try to correct the balance itself by building up flab in funny places: on thighs, in pads around the waist and hips, and even round the ankles. If you are weight-watching, it is often almost a 'mini-diet' simply to correct bad posture – suddenly, you look pounds slimmer. Holding in the stomach muscles properly when walking and sitting is particularly important for women; after childbearing, these muscles do lose tone and if you sag too much (or your stomach is artificially held in by tight jeans), they will develop into podgy, concertina-like mounds of flesh, with little or no muscular activity to encourage fat dispersal, and you will be stuck with a very podgy tum for a long time. During pregnancy, too, it is important to adjust the balance of your body to cope with the bump in front: tuck in your bottom, lifting the baby into the 'cradle' of your pelvis, walk tall and swing your arms. Do *not* lean back. Men, too, are guilty of the wobbly tummy problem – tuck it in! One way to check that you are walking well is to catch sight of yourself reflected in shop windows or on those TV monitor sets in stores. What a shock! Seriously, if you have ever seen a home movie or video, or even a photograph of yourself, you may realise only too well how bad your posture is.

Give yourself every chance of standing and walking well by making sure that you *carry* properly, and only what is strictly necessary. I try to carry as little as possible, and I think men do have the advantage of being less hampered by shopping than women. It is unfair! Get heavy loads delivered, and only carry the minimum. Two bags are better than one, for balance, taking the strain more evenly. Do not hunch or lean forward over whatever you are carrying; consciously relax your shoulders, and let your thigh muscles take the strain as they are supposed to. I have seen lots of schoolchildren carrying heavy bags of books over one shoulder, which makes me think we are due for a generation of people with one shoulder higher than the other; the old fashioned mode of a satchel on the back, or a couple of bags, would be a better idea. One fashion which does have my approval, though, is the female one for keeping a purse or bag on a strap *across* the body, from shoulder to hip. The weight is distributed much more evenly that way, and your arms are free to swing naturally while you walk. Never, ever 'put your back into' carrying anything.

Which brings me to the subject of lifting. Whether you are picking up a child, a bucket of

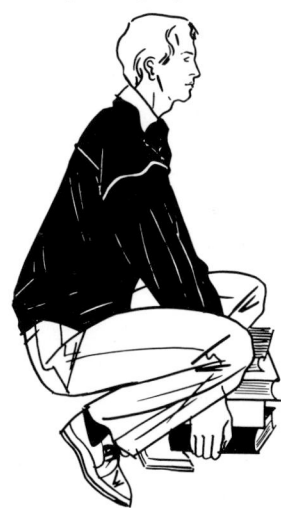

Take the strain on your thighs when lifting a heavy object, not on your back. Thigh muscles are usually underworked, and are tough enough to do this job, if you learn to use them.

water, a pile of books or whatever, you should always bend your knees and keep your spine straight. If you stoop, you will put undue strain on your back. Use the same rule when you are making beds, or getting something from a low shelf; bend those knees (they will creak at first, but the bones and muscles are very much more able to cope than the spine). You should also try to pull a heavy

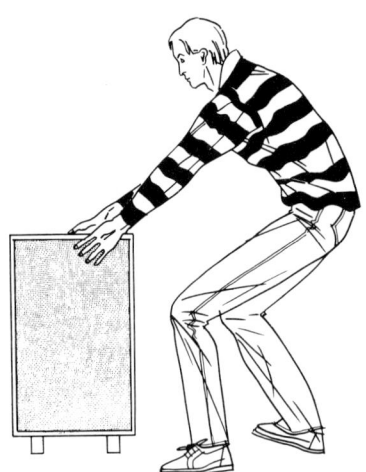
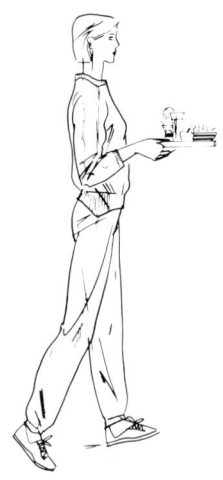

Pull a heavy object, rather than pushing it along, which can lead to back strain. Take the weight on your arms, legs.

Keep objects, such as trays, close to your body, so that they are easy to carry. Do not hunch over, and let your legs bear most of the strain.

object, rather than pushing it along, which inevitably causes strain. If you are holding something heavy like a tray of food, keep the object close to your body, rather than using outstretched arms. And remember to relax your shoulders and let your body and legs take the weight. This is really vital if you do a job where carrying is part of the action; if your shoulders and the muscles at the top of your spine are strained, you will find that you get nasty headaches as well as backache.

ENVIRONMENT

Everyday objects can also conspire to make your body become contorted. It seems crazy to make a big effort to improve your shape with exercise for an hour or so each day, when you spend a full eight hours sitting at a desk or work-bench which is the wrong height, giving you a permanent stoop. So, I suggest you take a good look at the objects which surround you and see if it is possible to improve the environment in which you have to function.

Cars

I have to drive many hundreds of miles each week to training sessions and events, and I have made sure that my car (a SAAB Turbo 900) is really comfort-

able. Although car seat design is said to be notoriously bad, I think individual requirements are so varied that it is impossible to rate one particular design above another. Slipped disc specialist Dr Bernard Watkins did attempt to give ratings, awarding stars (up to five for super) for firmness, thigh depth, shape, height, lumbar support. On that scale, only five cars – two Alfa Romeo models, one BMW model, the Range Rover and the Triumph Stag – were given four stars, and *no* car was rated five. Personally, I think you should test the car for your own needs when you buy it and adjust it where necessary.

The ideal seat should allow you to drive with your knees comfortably bent (not wedged up under the wheel), shoulders back and down, hands and arms relaxed, and back well supported, especially at the *lower* part which is particularly vulnerable to back pain. A small cushion placed behind your lower back can help here. Make sure you sit well back in the seat – if you hunch over the wheel on a long drive, the muscles in the back of your neck will become knotted, giving you an excruciating headache on arrival, and your stomach muscles will flop into Michelin-man folds, preventing that motorway meal from being digested properly.

Clear vision is also vital (it sounds obvious, but have you seen those idiots driving along peering over the wheel or attempting to see out of a filthy windscreen and completely obscured back window?) to prevent squint-lines appearing on your face, as well as for safety.

I hear a lot of complaints from drivers unused to wearing seat-belts, who have had to do so since it became law in Britain in January 1983. It could be well worth the expense of getting a new set fitted if you have a fairly old car which was fitted during manufacture. In the last few years, belts have become much more comfortable and easier to adjust, so that the passengers' shoulders are not dragged down. There really is no need to get shoulder ache.

Bicycles

Make sure your bike is comfortable as well as roadworthy. Do not ride around on a bike with the saddle too low, making you hunch. Your feet must be able to touch the ground when you are stationary (it is surprising how many children have to get off the saddle to stand at traffic lights). Make sure you check over saddle and handlebar heights regularly, especially if you are a fast-growing child or teenager.

Chairs

Ideally, when you sit at a table you should sit like this: well back, with buttocks pressed against the back of the chair, thighs pressed evenly on the seat, making a right angle with the lower part of your legs. Feet should be flat on the floor, with a 90° angle between feet and shins, backbone should be held upright (not stiffly, but in its natural curves), and shoulders should be back and down. The best kind of chair for long-term sitting should be straight-backed with good support at the lower-back. Swivel chairs are sometimes fine, but they do encourage flopping about, and sitting with legs at funny angles. A small cushion at the base of your spine is fine, but you should not sit on a cushion all day – the buttock muscles need something to brace *against* if they are to work properly: if they have nothing to contract against they simply give up and spread. That is why it is really better to watch TV sitting on a hard, high-backed chair, than all sprawled out on a squashy sofa. In fact, I prefer to sit on the floor with my bottom and back against the firm front of an armchair or sofa if I am listening to music or watching my video recordings. If I want to flop out, I would rather do it in bed than loll on a sofa. This makes sense, as the human body really is not designed for lolling.

Desks and tables

If you have to sit at a desk or a work-bench all day, choose a chair which allows you to sit with the surface at elbow-height so that you can work comfortably. If the desk is too high, you will get a stiff neck, if the desk is too low, your stomach will be pressed into a concertina shape and you will get very rounded shoulders. If you are on a factory production line, check that the stool or chair you sit on is not too high or too low for comfort – most bosses are fairly amenable when it comes to improving productivity, and you will find that you do work more efficiently if you are seated at the right height.

Work surfaces

A lot of thought goes into designing kitchen work-tops, boards in drawing offices and studios, and shop counters – but the vast majority of these are at the wrong height for comfort. Ideally, you should have surfaces at wrist-level when you are standing at them with elbows slightly bent, shoulders relaxed. Do a bit of adjustment by raising the level of your work, or lowering your own body with a stool. If the surface is too high, stand on a board or sit on a high stool to bring your body up to the most comfortable level. Migraine, sciatica and headaches are very common in offices and factories where work surfaces are the wrong height, and it seems daft to inflict these consequences on yourself in your own home.

Beds

A firm bed is definitely more comfortable and better for your body than a soft one. A well-sprung mattress will give more even support to muscles and limbs than a lumpy or sagging one. If you sink too far into your mattress with one part of your body, the other muscles have to work overtime to compensate, which can lead to aches and pains. Doctors say that going to bed drunk is one common cause of backache because the body is too doped to move around to ease cramped muscles. I think it is important to have plenty of room in bed, too, so that you can have a good stretch. Do not have soft mounds of pillows; they make you hunch your shoulders and can cause double chins.

I am very interested in the whole subject of beds as I do spend a lot of my time sleeping – around nine hours a night. One great bonus of taking plenty of exercise is that insomnia is hardly ever a problem – quite the opposite! People who ring me at 9.30 a.m. are often surprised not only to find me in (I do not go running until about 9.45 a.m.), but also actually tucked up in bed. I know that is impossible for most people, but I really do recommend that you improve the *quality* of your sleep if not the quantity, by checking that you are getting the very best service from your bedding.

Lighting

Lighting does not actually shape your body, but it does affect your health more dramatically than you are probably aware. I am lucky in that I get *my* 'industrial' lighting from the sun itself because my work is mainly outside. If you do work indoors, however, you need your work adequately lit – there are strict rules about that – and you also need good quality lighting. It is now known that the popular fluorescent-type of lighting can be harmful because it distorts the natural light in several ways leading to visual difficulties and even skin problems. The 'full spectrum' type of lighting is closest to natural light, and although it is more expensive than the ordinary fluorescent type, I think it is worth it. Tests in American schools have shown that pupils work better, feel less droopy and are less often absent from school, under this type of lighting.

Whatever the type you use, do make sure that you do not have to squint to do your work; the work itself, not your head or face, should be well-lit. When you are watching TV, never sit in the dark concentrating like mad on the goggle-box, and do make sure that the set is properly adjusted; you quickly get used to a fuzzy picture or 'bleeding' colour edges, but your eyesight will be seriously harmed. And bad eyesight can in turn affect your general posture.

YOU HAVE ONLY ONE BODY – MAKE THE MOST OF IT!

It is your body – but do you know how it works? As a top athlete, I have had to make a close study of human anatomy, and it makes sense for everyone to know as much as possible about the workings of his or her own body. Here is a guide to the major muscle groups, and the types of exercise and sports which help keep them healthy:

MAJOR MUSCLE GROUPS

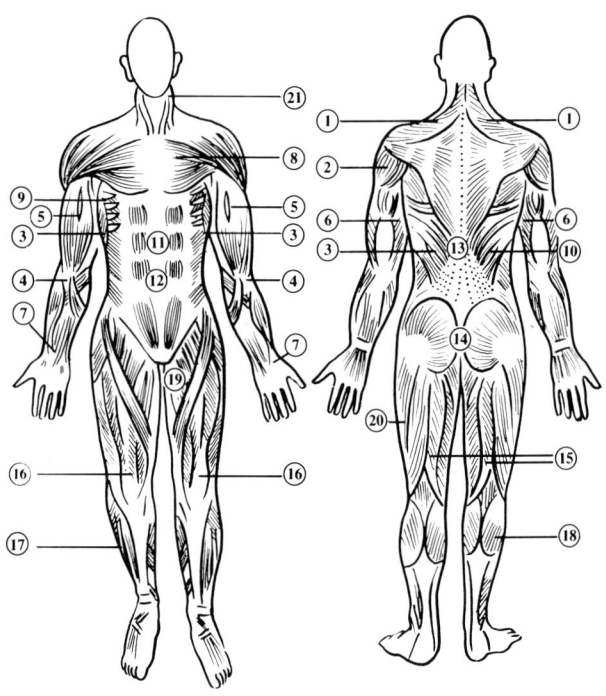

1 Trapezius: Triangular shaped muscle across the back of the neck and shoulders.
This draws the shoulders together and downwards. Bad tone can make your shoulders rounded and painful. Very susceptible to strain.
Exercise by shoulder-circling, backward arm swings (pp. 63, 64).
2 Deltoids: These stretch over the top of the shoulders covering the shoulder joints.
These raise up the arms to shoulder level, sidewards, and work with other muscles to help rotate arms and raise them front and back.
Exercise by arm-raising (p. 36) or weightlifting (p. 67), gymnastics, climbing, boxing, tennis (p. 100).
3 Latissimus dorsi: This is a broad muscle, stretching across the back into the backs of the arms.
This draws arms down and back and rotates them.
Exercise by pulling arms down and backwards (p. 49), and sports like rowing, climbing ('chinning' on p. 100).
4 Brachialis: Stretch across the fronts of the upper arms, across the joints.
They help to flex the arms in conjunction with the biceps.
Exercise by arm-bending against resistance with weights (p. 80), digging the garden.
5 Biceps: Fronts of the upper arms.

They turn hands palm upwards to bend the arms.
Exercise with weights (p. 75).

6 Triceps: Backs of the upper arms.
They straighten the elbows.
Exercise by pushing arms against resistance (p. 48), sports like cricket, baseball, javelin, boxing.

7 Wrist flexors: Fronts of the forearms.
They help bend the palms of the hands towards you.
Exercise by hand-gripping (p. 49), pushing wrists forwards, sports like golf (p. 103), bowls, squash, badminton.

8 Pectorals: Upper chest, above the breasts.
They help to draw the arms across the body, and rotate arms inwards. They do a useful job helping to support the breasts.
Should be given a daily 'workout' for this reason. Exercise by pushing against an immovable object (p. 49), grabbing your wrists and pushing hard.

9 Serratus anterior: Sides of the upper ribcage.
They help you push with your arms.
Push against resistance to exercise them (p. 49), or mow the lawn, sweep the carpet, push a pram.

10 Intercostals: Between the ribs in two layers.
They help you breathe, by raising and lowering the ribs as you inhale and exhale.
Breathing exercises (p. 18).

11 Abdominals: Group forming a muscular 'corset' three layers thick between diaphragm and pelvis.
They bend the trunk from side to side, support the stomach – or do not depending on how well they work. Most sports involve some abdominal work.
Exercise with 'sit up' movements (p. 35), dancing (p. 83).

12 Rectus abdominis: Extend down the middle of the abdominals to the pubic bone.
They bend the trunk forwards.
Exercise by bending forward (p. 88), golf, rowing, leg-raises (p. 37).

13 Erector spinae: Extend the whole length of the spinal column.
They help the spine to move smoothly, keep the trunk erect.
Exercise by back-arching movements, raising the trunk from forward position (pp. 26–28, 40).

14 Buttock group: Extend all over the seat.
They pull thighs sideways, backwards, move the legs, some help raise the trunk from a stooping position.
Exercise by contraction (p. 50), raising legs backwards (p. 40).

15 Hamstring group: Rear of the thighs.
They bend knees, help them rotate outwards, extend legs backwards. Vulnerable because they do not get enough use.
Toe touching and leg stretching exercises can help (pp. 36, 65, 104–106).

16 Quadriceps femoris: Fronts of thighs.
They extend the knees, bend the hips.
Leg straightening and kicking movements are good (pp. 34, 37) plus soccer (p. 92), running (p. 59).

17 Tibialis anterior: Fronts of lower legs
They raise toes and feet up and towards you, turn feet inwards.
Exercise by foot bending, circling, turning feet up (pp. 50, 65).

18 Calves group: Backs of lower legs.
They raise heels, point toes downwards.
Heel raising, toe pointing, walking, running (p. 59), dancing (p. 83).

19 Adductors: Insides of thighs.
They pull upper legs inwards.
Riding, swimming (p. 107), squeezing ankles against resistance (p. 48).

20 Abductors: Outside of thighs.
They carry legs outwards and rotate them inwards.
Walking and running with feet pointing forwards is good exercise (p. 59).

21 Sternomastoid: Each side of the neck.
These act independently to bend the head sideways and turn it, and act together to bend the head on to the chest.
Exercise by head bending, head rotation (p. 63).

TAKE A BREATHER!

Are you breathing properly? One of the (many!) advantages of taking exercise is that it helps increase your breathing efficiency. Most of us take the whole process very much for granted until we study our respiratory system in more detail. Did you know, for instance, that if our two lungs were spread flat, with all the wrinkles ironed out, they would cover an area equal to that of half a tennis court? Neither did I, until I became an athlete and had to monitor my own breathing processes. Because our lungs have this super capacity, they are capable of the most tremendous performance which is rarely demanded in everyday life. Most people use only minimum lung capacity in general breathing, and could improve the way they feel and their general health with better breathing.

Why? Because the oxygen which we breathe in is very useful stuff indeed – once it has dissolved on the moist lining of the lungs and passed through the walls into the red cells of the blood, it is carried first to the heart and then to all the tissues of the body. It is used by our bodily cells to break down food substances, particularly sugar, to set free the energy stored in it. This breaking down of foods is the essential part of the whole respiratory process – no cell can work unless it has energy, and it can only get this energy from food if the breaking-down process takes place. So, do not just think of 'energy' as something you have when you feel full of get-up-and-go; it is actually something which is working at all times on all bodily cells – including those of the brain!

What happens when we breathe?

Well, one layer of muscles between the ribs contracts, lifting them upwards and outwards, making the cavity wider. The lower ribs move most, rather like the handle of a bucket, when you raise it from resting to half way up. The muscles of the diaphragm contract, making it flatter and making the chest cavity longer. It pushes on the abdominal organs so that the front of the abdominal wall bulges a little. As the walls and chest floor move out, the lungs are pulled outwards, too, and as they become larger, the pressure falls . . . and air is pushed into the body to cope, via the nose and air passages. A different layer of muscles between the ribs now takes over, pulling the ribs back down and inwards, squashing the lungs so that the air is forced out again.

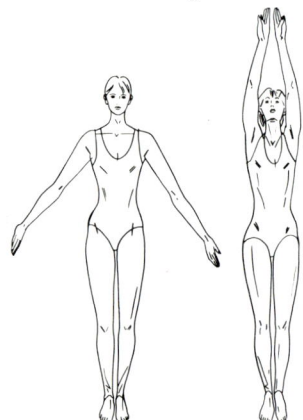

The Complete Breath

To find out just how efficient breathing *feels*, try this yoga exercise. It is a good one to use before an important interview or when you have spent hours cooped up in a stuffy train or plane and want to feel terrific. It is also a good choice if you enjoy deep breathing in front of an open window in the morning.

1 Stand with your back straight, head erect and legs and feet together, with hands hanging loosely down.
2 Now inhale deeply, at the same time bringing your arms slowly up at the sides, with the palms uppermost.

3 Let the backs of your hands touch above your head.
4 Exhale as you lower the arms back down to your sides, but do not rush, just let the air gently come out through your mouth.
5 Repeat eight times.

Aerobics

There has been a lot of publicity given to aerobic exercises, as if they were something new and revolutionary. In fact, the term simply means 'with oxygen' and it is used to describe any exercises which demand oxygen without causing an intolerable oxygen debt, which means that they can be continued for long periods: dancing, jogging, doing rapid exercises to music – they are all 'aerobics'. Tennis does not really count because you stop for a breather every time a point is scored, and football is equally erratic.

'Anaerobic' exercises ('without oxygen') fall into two categories: the kind which demand reasonable amounts of oxygen but are cut short voluntarily (like running for a short distance or doing a short workout with breaks between exercises); and the kind which demand so much oxygen that you *have* to stop because your heart and lungs cannot cope otherwise – things like very fast sprints, bicycle sprints, dashing for the bus, all come into that category.

In this book, you will be trying both aerobic and anaerobic (the first kind only, we do not intend to wear you out!) exercises, and isometrics too (explanation of *that* term in chapter 6).

Going back to aerobics, you should beware of trying a frantic, rapid exercise-to-music workout unless you are ready for it – which means that you are used to long, sustained effort. Do not try to leap into an aerobics class, hooked on the jargon about pulse rates, if your body cannot cope. You may well slow your pulse rate down, but you are also likely to slow down your whole body: I am more in favour of using pulse rate measurement as an *occasional* early morning check-up to find out whether, in fact, your exercising efforts are helping to slow things down nicely. As someone who is just getting into shape, your resting pulse rate is likely to be 75–80 beats a minute. Once you start a regular exercise programme, this could slow down to about 60 beats a minute. A marathon runner I met once had a resting rate of only 32 beats a minute. My own resting pulse rate is about 48–50, unless I am feeling twitchy.

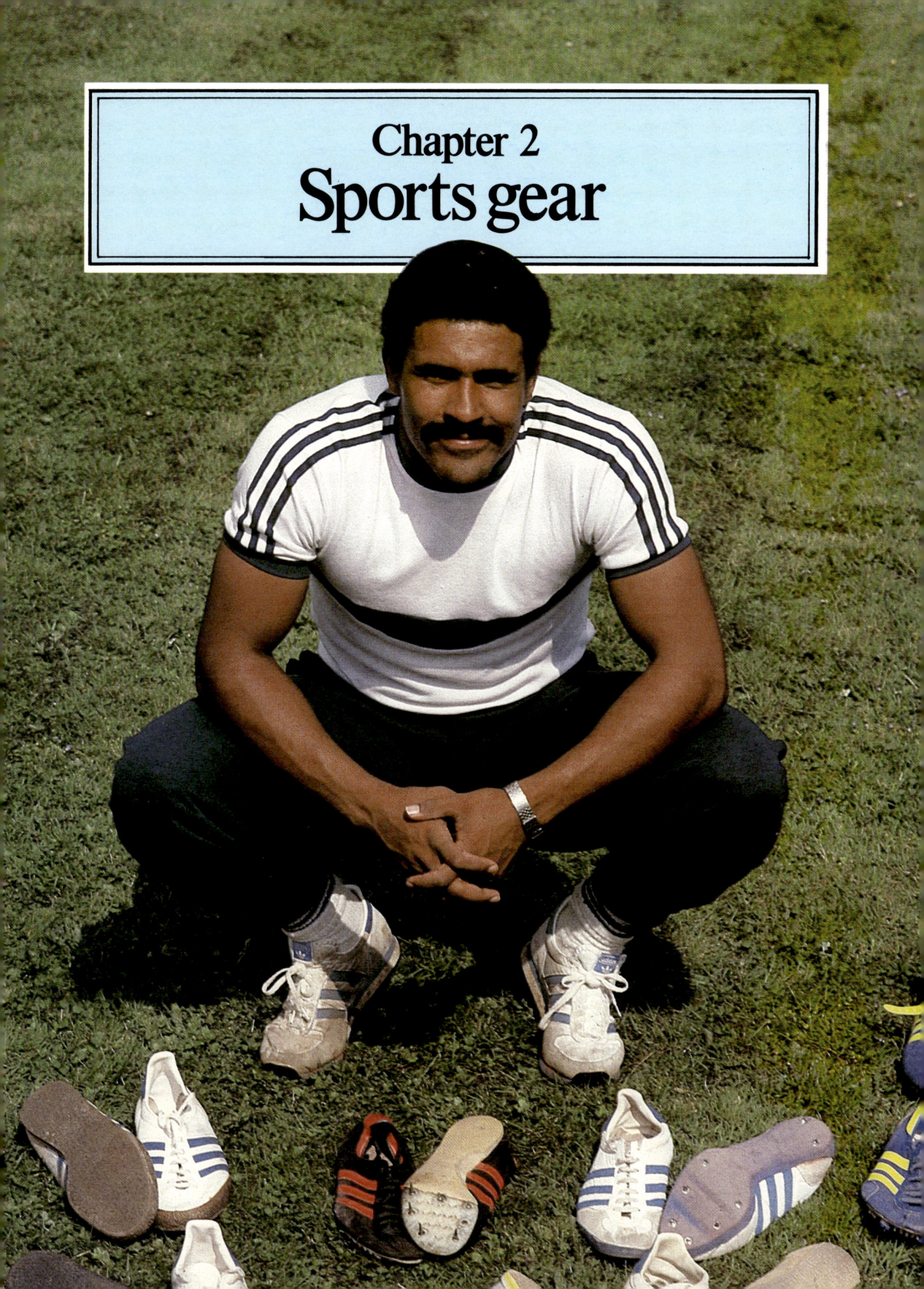

Chapter 2
Sports gear

Sport should be fun, and if you choose the right gear – and look after it properly – you will enjoy your sport more, as well as derive a real psychological advantage by being well turned out.

FOOTWEAR

Running shoes

There are now about 180 different types of running shoe available on the British market. Many of them include special women's versions, which are narrower at the heel and instep and made in smaller sizes and prettier colours. But, really, colour is the last thing you should worry about. Remember that, if you are a keen runner, your shoes have to take the shock of about 800 footfalls per mile, the equivalent of 61 tonnes (60 tons) per foot per mile for a 63 kg (10 stone) runner.

Modern shoes are divided into three sections – sole, mid-sole and upper, and it is the mid-sole area where most of the research has been carried out by big companies like Adidas and Nike. That is where the shock-absorption factor is incorporated into the design – usually using a substance called Ethylene Vinyl Acetate, a polymer material which has bubbles of air trapped in it. The actual sole itself is usually made of either solid rubber (longer-lasting for distance runners), or the lighter, bouncier 'blown' rubber. Choose a wavy, flat sole for road-jogging or training; a studded waffle sole for rough ground if you enjoy jogging through open country like me; or the newer cantilever type sole, which has super shock-absorption and decreases injury risk. The shoe's upper is likely to be made of a quick-drying lightweight synthetic, with leather or suede trim. It is very important that the stitching *inside* the upper does not rub or irritate your foot – vulnerable points are around the lacing and heel. Very high-backed shoes can be a problem too – the stiff heel-tab may rub the back of your ankle making it sore.

When you are buying shoes, do go to a specialist shop where the assistants are sports fans and know what they are talking about. Go in the afternoon, when your feet are likely to be a bit swollen, wearing the socks you will wear with the shoes. You may find that you need a shoe a half or even a whole size larger than your normal shoe size. Walk, or even

run, around the shop a few times before you decide.

You can test your own feet for flexibility by doing the bathmat test. Sit on the side of the bath and make a footprint on the mat. Now stand up and make another print. If it is the same size or only slightly larger than the first print, your feet are rigid and need well-cushioned shoes. If it is much larger, your feet are more flexible, so look for a snug heel fit and good arch support.

You can also look at the soles of a pair of old jogging shoes to check whether you are 'pronating' or not. 'Pronators' are runners whose feet turn inward, or pronate, as they hit the ground. Although most of us do this, if the movement becomes exaggerated it can lead to injury – particularly to shins and knees. If you are an 'extreme pronator', the inside edge and heel of your shoe will be well worn down, and the main area of wear on the ball of your foot will be on the inside. There are shoes available which can counteract this effect by supporting your feet to prevent that inward roll. But you should check with your doctor or club physio if this is a real problem.

If all this sounds a bit specialised to someone who goes jogging a few times a week in battered 'trainers', I can only say try jogging in decent shoes and see how much more fun it is. This advice is particularly important for youngsters with developing feet; if you do a cross-country stint every week at school, you *must* keep checking your shoes for comfort and fit, and if you like to kick a ball around and play hectic games at weekends, you really do need to choose footwear carefully. Try to save up for good shoes, please!

Soccer boots

Because I am a keen footballer, my soccer boots are very well looked after and they are good ones. If you are buying, go for leather if possible. Your boots should be very supple (one test is to bend the uppers right back – they should almost bend in *half*) with screw-in studs which can be changed to suit the conditions of the pitch. Nylon studs which are allowed to wear down can become very sharp and dangerous, and the rubber type may feel comfy, but they really are not practical unless the surface is dry and grassless. Choose a pair with a long tongue to protect your ankles, and well-fitted heels for support. They should fit well – it is not really a good investment to buy a youngster boots which are too big, because he will not be able to play properly, and they may even be a hazard if they slide about. Look after soccer boots by allowing them to dry naturally (*not* in your sports bag), cleaning them thoroughly, and polishing regularly with a good shoe polish. Get repairs done quickly.

Tennis shoes

Like running shoes, these should be tried on carefully before purchase – allow yourself plenty of time. Choose a pair with ample arch support, and uppers which are cut comfortably so that they do not cause blistering or soreness around the ankle. If you have heel protectors on your shoes, make sure they are the cushioned type, which will not irritate the Achilles tendon. When you try on the shoes, do not lace them too tightly, and take a pair of sports socks with you to gauge the proper fit.

Sports socks

Most youngsters these days seem to pick the cushioned type of sports sock in Orlon or another synthetic material. These are fine, as long as the seaming is neat (raised seams can chafe badly), and they are the correct size. Never wear too-tight socks, and make sure you have plenty of pairs available so that you can always change into a fresh, dry pair when necessary. Some people swear by natural fibres only for socks, but pure cotton or cotton and wool mixture can sometimes become hard with constant washing, and it tends to hold perspiration more. Synthetic mixtures dry quickly and do not need such careful rinsing, although you should still make sure that you do give them a thorough rinse. Use soap flakes instead of detergent – lots of people are allergic to detergent, which can give sensitive feet nasty sores.

Exercise tights

These should be long enough in the leg to allow maximum movement. Ideally, wear footless tights for exercise, as they allow full flexibility, and you are less likely to slip in your bare feet or wearing shoes than you would in 'stockinged feet'.

CLOTHING

Shorts and leotards

While I would prefer anyone to take exercise wearing jeans and a jumper rather than take none at all, I firmly believe that comfortable clothes designed for the job are much better. You cannot run properly or play tennis if your stomach is constricted, so look for shorts which fit neatly round the hips, but are roomy around the waistline and legs. Make sure tops tuck well in so that you do not come apart around the middle, and have roomy shoulders and sleeves so that you can swing your arms properly and make those superb overhead shots. If you wear a leotard for your dance class, choose one which is long enough, from neckline to crutch, to let you move properly without straining or feeling cut in two. The very strong Lycra type of leotard looks good, but can restrict circulation and cause muscle cramps if you try to squeeze too much flesh into it. The sleeves are often very narrow indeed – be careful that your hands do not become numb because your circulation has been restricted above the elbow.

Tracksuits

This is a subject close to my heart – and almost every other part of my anatomy because I spend most of my time wearing tracksuits of one kind or another. I like the type with a roomy, comfortable trouser waistband, and zip pockets so that valuables stay secure when I am running or working out. The latest designs are so fashionable that I am not surprised that people wear them for all kinds of activities as well as for sport. Remember that the real purpose of a tracksuit is to keep you warm before and after an event, which means you need one with a good fleecy lining for the British winter and you should make sure that the top is long enough to keep draughts out. I find the nylon type too sweaty for comfort and prefer synthetic mixtures containing cotton – but nylon is certainly quick-drying if you like to jog or play tennis in all weathers. There is a very important psychological advantage in jumping into a tracksuit when you get up in the morning – you feel sporty, so you act that way. Put on a tracksuit to do the housework or go for a walk, and you will soon find yourself being brisk and energetic.

Underwear

Underwear to be worn for all sport and exercise should be cool and absorbent in cotton or cotton and synthetic mixture. For men, the fashion for wearing cotton briefs instead of a jockstrap is fine, so long as the briefs are well-cut with a wide crotch which cannot cut into you. Shorts with built-in pants can be uncomfortable because the pants are synthetic, and jockstraps to get a bit saggy with constant washing. For women, cotton pants are best or at least synthetic with a cotton gusset. This is particularly important under a synthetic leotard, where chafing and lack of absorbency can encourage uncomfortable soreness and even infection.

As for bras, well, I have never actually suffered from 'jogger's nipple', but I have heard that it can be very painful! It is caused by chafing when a bra-less lady's breast or man's chest rubs against her or his vest or sweater. If you are a lady of size 75 (34″) or over you should really wear a bra, otherwise your breasts will feel heavy and the pectoral muscles which support them will be stretched. My lady sporting friends tell me that there are some excellent sports bras on the market with seamless cups and wide shoulder straps to take the strain. Keep your bra straps adjusted for comfort, but do not make them too tight or you will feel a real pull on shoulder muscles during most sporting activities which will mess up your performance and give you nasty neck twinges.

What about thermal underwear? Wear it in winter by all means – I always wear warm tights under my shorts or tracksuit in winter. If your legs are cold, they are more likely to become stiff or injured. Muscles need to be warm to relax, to avoid cramp and to function at their maximum efficiency. For this reason, leg warmers are also a good idea in exercise class. Outdoors wear gloves, a hat and a long-sleeved T-shirt, too, if you are at all chilly.

Waterproofs

It is not really comfortable to run in bulky waterproofs, but a new fabric called Gore-tex has recently come on the market which is lightweight *and* waterproof, and actually allows you to perspire properly by allowing perspiration to evaporate. This is excellent for golfers, walking fans, and hardy joggers – but it is expensive.

Swimwear

The newest swimwear is light and very streamlined indeed, but, quite frankly, you do not need anything really special for swimming as long as it is comfortable. If you are a really keen swimmer, though, look at the professional styling of competitive swimwear – you will find that it has the super cut and fit you need, plus, of course, the 'go faster' stripes to make you feel speedy. Shoulder strap design is important for ladies: the halter kind of fastening is rarely comfortable – you need built-in shoulder straps which fit snugly without being too tight. Try nude swimming if you can one day – it really is a sensational feeling. Women who have indulged in topless swimming find that they enjoy the feeling of freedom, but I only recommend this if you have a small, perfect bustline and the natives are friendly.

Safety wear

Despite the pleas of the Royal Society for the Prevention of Accidents, many joggers and cyclists still go around at night in dark sweaters and trousers. Wear white, or, better still, get yourself fixed up with the most visible type of bib or armbands in 3M Scotchlite, made up of tiny reflective beads which pick up the lights from car headlamps. Fluorescent tops are good too, but old, well-washed ones are not so effective as new ones and really cannot be relied upon to give you instant visibility in total blackness. Carry a small torch, too, for extra insurance, and be sensible about where you jog or cycle at night.

TENNIS, SQUASH AND BADMINTON RACQUETS

For *all* specialist sporting equipment, I strongly advise trying out various makes, weights and styles before you buy. You must go along to a good sports department or store, and have a chat with the experts on hand. In my experience, they do not try to sell you the most expensive products, and they do give good advice. It is not a good idea for parents to buy sports equipment for their child as a surprise; far better to get him or her fitted out properly on the spot.

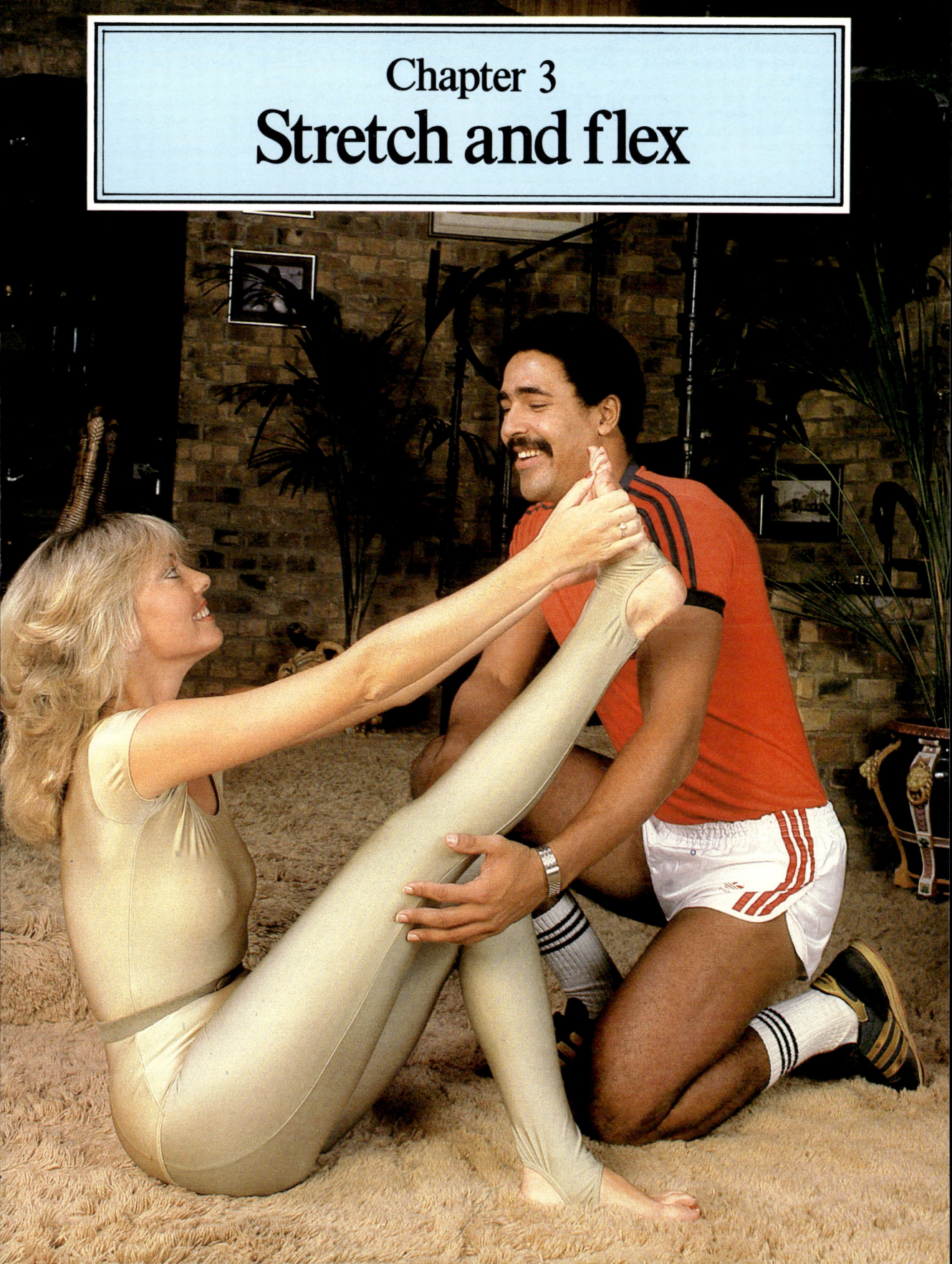

Chapter 3
Stretch and flex

Before you start any sort of exercise programme, or think of getting involved in a sport, it is a good idea to test your body for flexibility. Many people make the mistake of plunging straight into a fairly strenuous workout without being certain that their muscles are flexible enough to cope with the movements involved – quite apart from the potential danger to heart, lungs and blood pressure. Even if you are youngish and have a strong heart, do not smoke and never put salt on your food, the fact that you spend most of your time hunched up in an office or car may well mean that your body is less able to cope than you think. Try these simple tests:

1 While standing, can you pick up an object (something small) from the ground without bending your knees?
2 Can you sit on a sofa with one leg tucked under you, back straight, in perfect comfort?
3 Can you sit on your heels with your feet stretched out?
4 Now, can you bend forward and touch the ground with your forehead without raising your bottom from your heels?
5 Can you sit cross-legged – and then get up without using your hands?

No? I must admit that I cannot do 1 either – but all the others are easy! Seriously, those few movements will simply demonstrate to you how tense your muscles probably are – and this can even be true if you play some kind of sport, like soccer, fairly regularly. For, in many cases, sports place the emphasis less on flexibility and far more on strength, skill and endurance. The result can be overtense muscles which are more susceptible to injury, soreness and cramp.

If your muscles are tight, there is unnecessary pressure on blood capillaries, which may prevent oxygen from reaching the body cells properly, which in turn could limit your performance, especially where endurance is concerned. This means that you find yourself huffing and puffing by half-time or asking for a rest after 15 minutes of a 45-minute workout class.

So, I think it is really essential to do regular warm-up exercises with the emphasis on promoting flexibility. I suggest using two kinds of exercise: rhythmic exercises, which are swinging and rotational movements, and include such activities as skipping, arm-swinging, running on the spot; and static stretching exercises, which are very simple,

controlled movements often based on yoga poses. The idea is to perform the movement as accurately as possible, without strain, working towards 'perfection' if possible, but never overdoing things. The static stretching exercises are also useful for 'unwinding' your body after a day spent sitting at a desk. If you are feeling tired and irritable, they will also calm you down (that useful oxygen boost again) and get you into an optimistic mood for the evening – whether you are off to a disco or about to do battle for the honours in a club squash tournament match.

Always perform flexibility exercises in a warm environment or wearing warm clothing if you are outside and the weather is chilly. Warmth really does maximise all the benefits of flexibility exercises – in fact, it is dangerous to perform any of these exercises when your body is cold. I am strongly in favour of warmth and comfort whenever possible!

RHYTHMIC EXERCISES

Skipping

This is great fun, and the perfect rhythmic flexibility exercise. It also has the advantage of taking up very little room – many athletes and fitness fans find that their skipping rope is the most useful piece of equipment they can pack. Wear light, comfortable clothes, and flexible shoes. Try to think of your feet as feathers when you skip – if you come down on them too hard you could hurt them. Use a proper skipping rope with ball-bearing handles if possible. Grip the handles firmly, hands and forearms back so that they are at right angles, straight out at the sides, with hands at waist-level, rope resting behind your heels.

Start with a simple running step, turning the rope rhythmically and running in place with no bounce in between. Keep it up for a minute, then rest; then try another minute.

Gradually perfect the step, getting those knees higher, and aiming to stay in one place instead of wandering about. Increase your skipping time to five minutes or more – but do not overdo it. At the end of the session, do the Complete Stretch exercise (page 29).

As you become more proficient, try these steps:

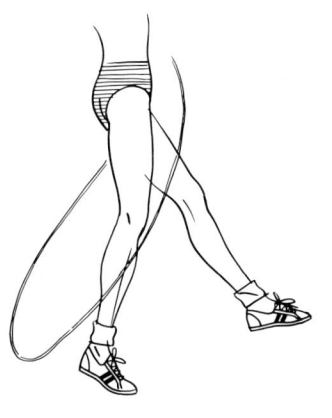
Rest Step

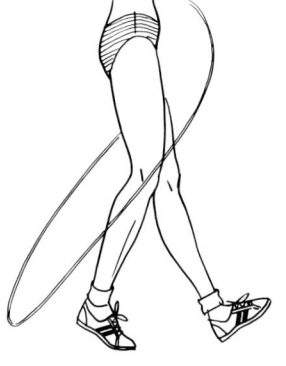
Heel Taps

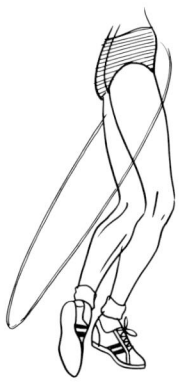
Crossovers

1 REST STEP

Jump over the rope, landing on the ball of your right foot. As the rope is turning, bounce again on that foot with a little hop, kicking the left foot out. Now land on the ball of your left foot and repeat.

2 HEEL TAPS

Jump on to the ball of your right foot, tapping your left heel on the floor out in front of you. Now jump on to the ball of your left foot, tapping your right heel out in front of you. Repeat.

3 CROSSOVERS

Land on the ball of your right foot, kicking your left leg back behind the right leg. Now land on the ball of your left foot and repeat, keeping your knees bent.

You can also try skipping games with a group or your family:

1 JUMPING IN

Skip with a long rope, and let your partner jump in, skipping with you, facing you. After ten steps, he or she must jump out again, and another partner takes a turn.

2 LONG ROPE GAMES

Get two people to turn a long rope and let each of the other members of the group jump in for ten turns each. If one member 'fluffs' his turn – then he is 'out'. It makes things even more difficult if the 'turners' use two ropes instead of one.

Arm, hand and shoulder exercises

'Lock' your fingers and rotate your wrists clockwise and then anti-clockwise for a few seconds. Now turn your palms outwards, but keep your fingers locked while you swing your arms overhead, as high as possible, then back down. Extend the arms straight in front of you, swing from side to side. Now stretch them overhead again, and swing to the right, then the left. Do five swings in each position, increasing to ten.

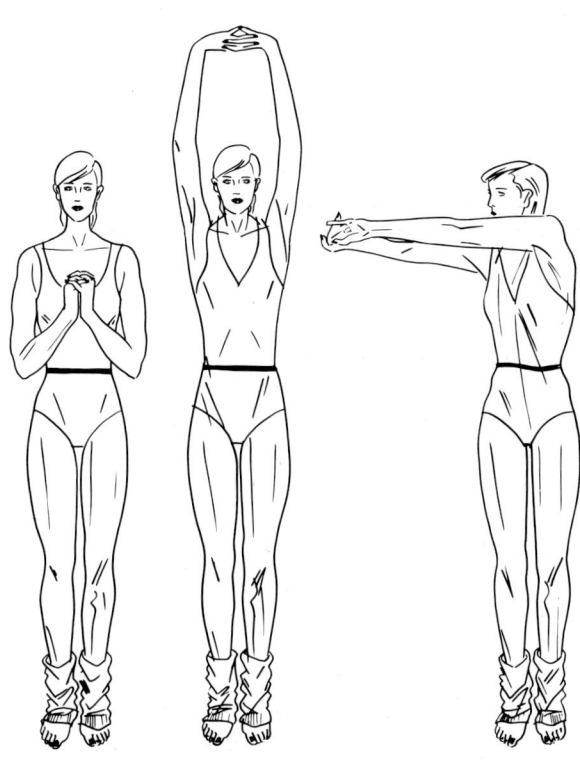

Lunge stretches

Stand, with right leg forward, left leg back, legs wide apart and straight. Raise arms above your head. Keeping your back straight, bend your right knee, taking the weight forward with your hips. Now straighten up and repeat five times increasing to ten. Repeat with left leg forward.

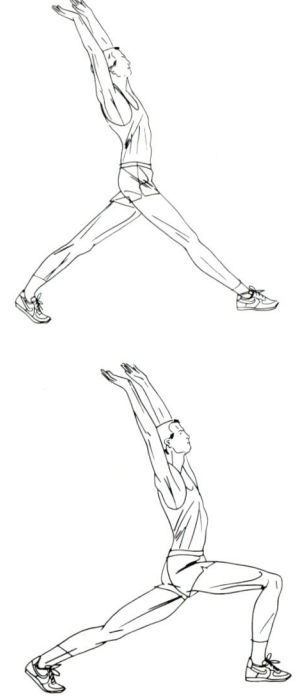

STATIC STRETCHING EXERCISES

These take up very little room, and are ideal for after work.

1 For back, legs, arms, stomach muscles
Stand, feet together, arms above your head, fingers clasped loosely. Look up at your hands. Bend your knees and bring your hands down slowly to the horizontal position, with your knees bent. Let your hands fall sideways and down, and relax your head forward. Pause, then reverse the movement. Repeat five times. Breathe in as you raise your body, out as you lower it.

2 For hamstrings, feet
Sit on the floor, back straight, knees bent, feet flat. Now grasp the ball of your left foot with both hands and lift it off the floor. Straighten leg as much as possible (do not strain) without curving your back or letting go of your foot. Repeat five times with each leg.

3 For thighs and hip mobility
Sit on the floor, hands behind you for support, back straight, knees bent. Now swing your hips to the left, lowering both knees to touch the floor. Repeat to the right. Repeat complete movement, right and left, five times.

4 For spine, shoulder and neck muscles
Kneel on the floor, and place your hands on the floor in front of you with hands shoulders' width apart. Knees should be together, feet stretched out (do not push your toes into the floor). Now hollow your back, head up. Hold for a count of five, then arch your back, letting your head hang down. Count five and repeat five times.

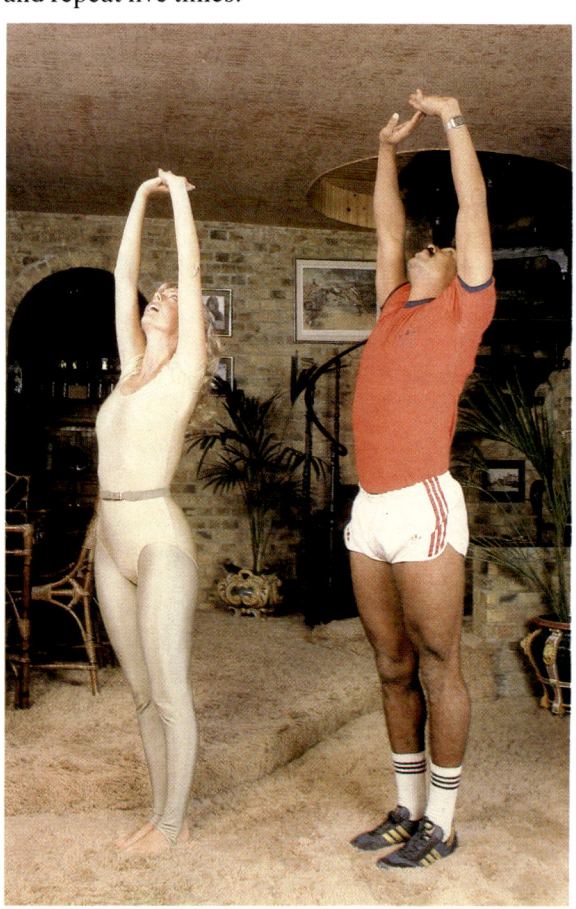

1a For back, legs, arms, stomach muscles

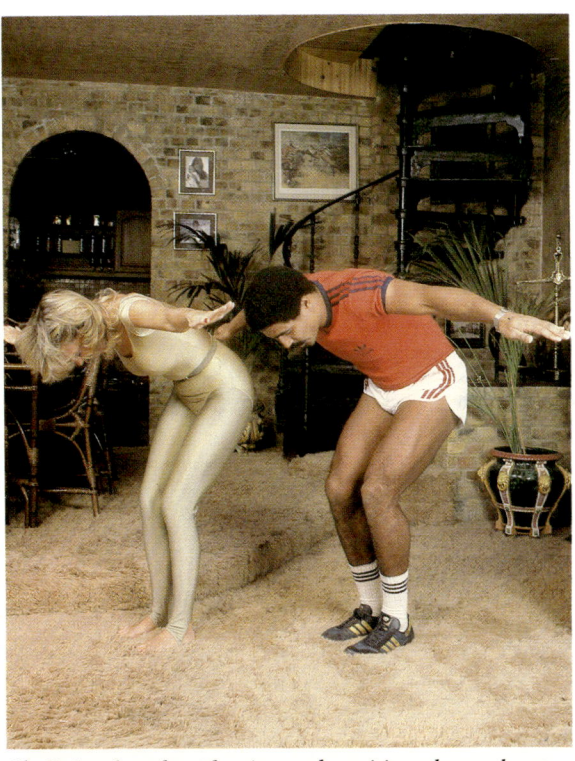

1b Bring hands to horizontal position, knees bent.

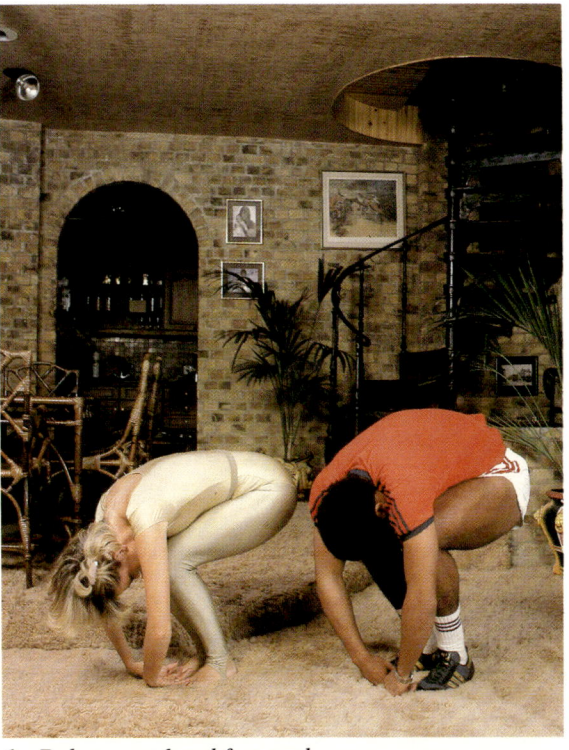

1c Relax your head forward

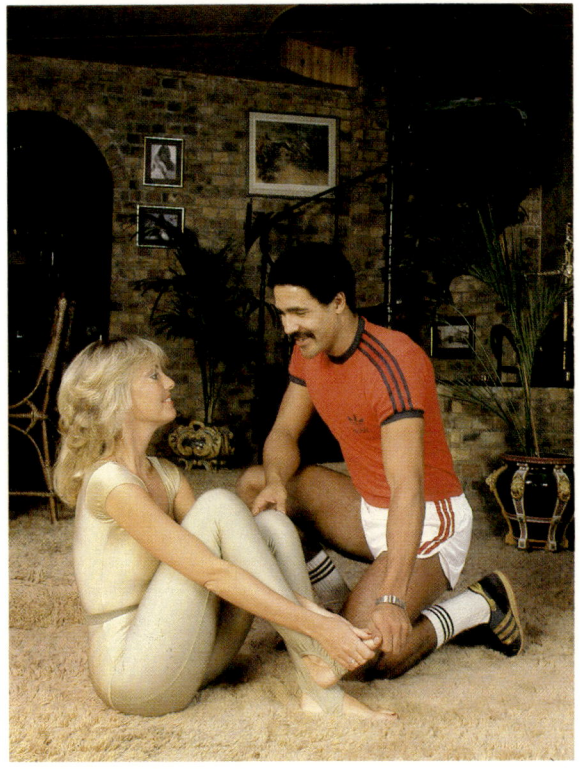

2 For hamstrings, feet

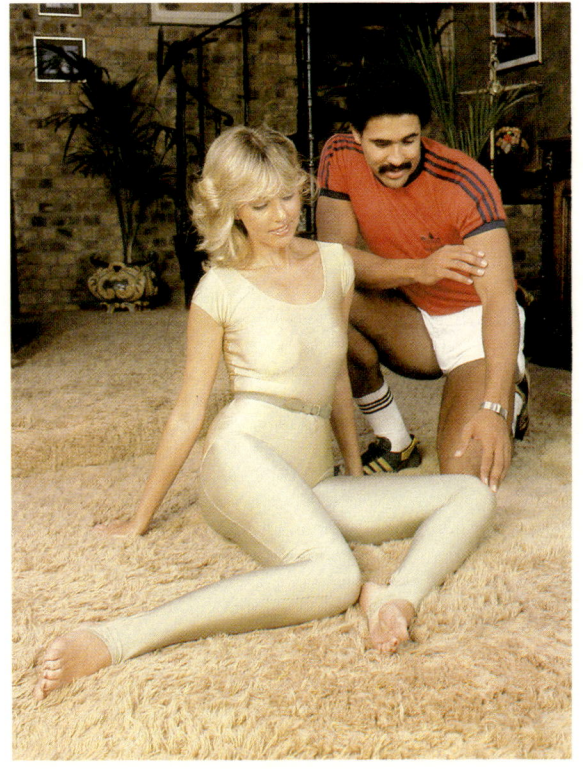

3 For thighs and hip mobility

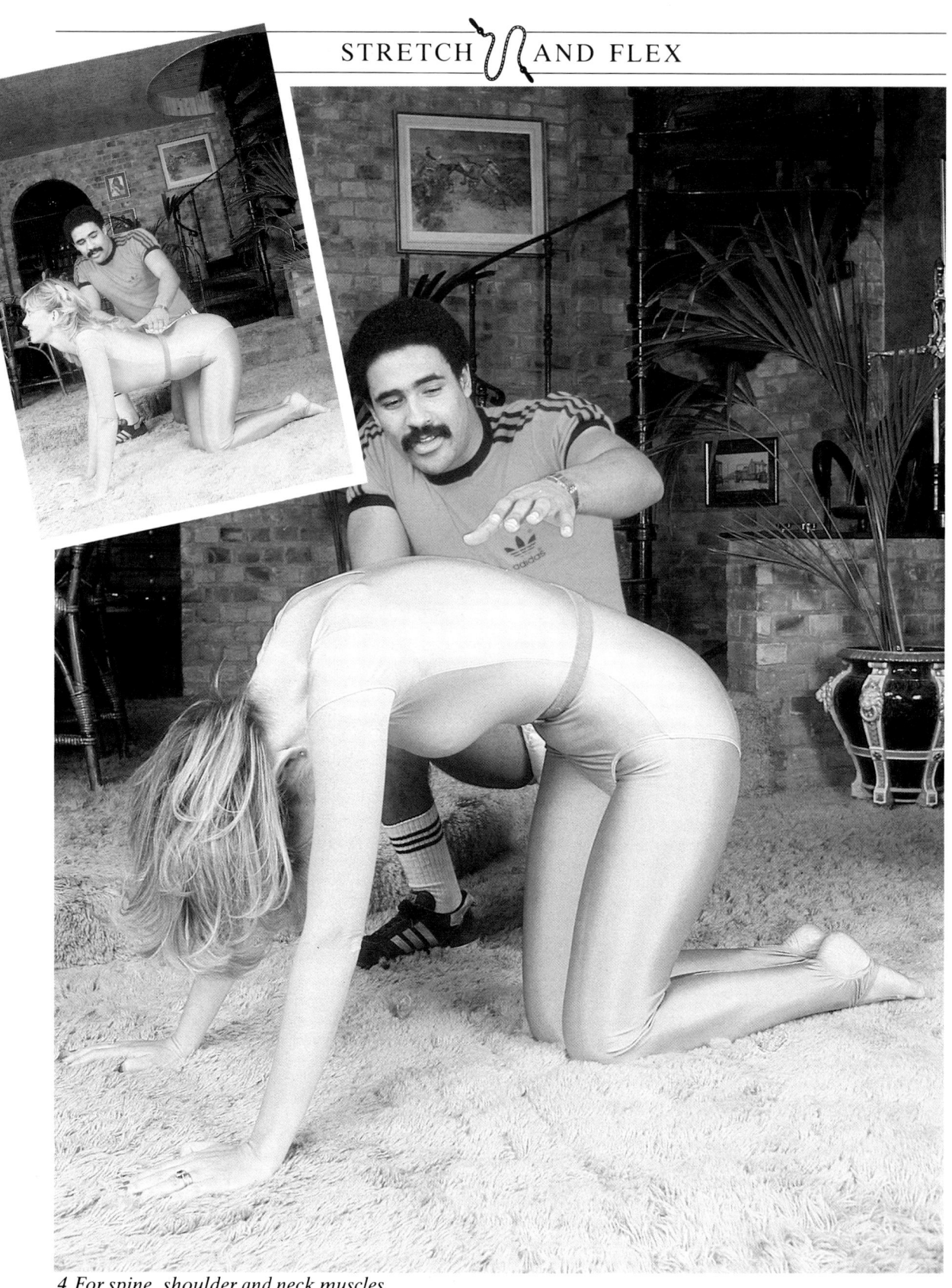

4 For spine, shoulder and neck muscles

Complete stretch

Lie on your back, feet slightly apart, hands by your sides with palms uppermost. Let your feet flop apart and breathe slowly and rhythmically for a few seconds. Now stretch your right arm above your head, your right leg down, pointing the toe as hard as you can. Repeat twice, then repeat with your left arm and leg. Roll over on to your stomach, legs and feet together, hands by your sides palms uppermost. Let your chin rest on the floor. Bend your knees, letting your feet come in towards your bottom. Reach back with your hands and hold your feet. Keep your elbows straight and start to raise your head. Gently push your feet back towards the floor, pulling your shoulders back, and raise your chin to look at the ceiling. Hold for a count of five, then relax. Repeat once only. This is a superb stretching movement for the whole body.

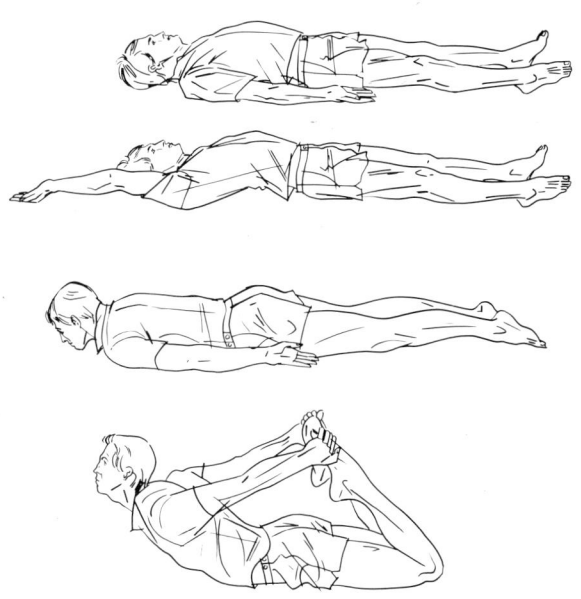

Standing leg grip

Stand with your legs and feet about 60 cm (2′) apart, and relax forwards from the waist, with head and hands hanging down, elbows straight. Take a deep breath in through the nose. Now grip your legs and raise your head slightly, keeping your elbows straight. Exhale. Pull on your legs, letting your elbows go out to your sides, and bringing your head in as far as you can. Count five, and let your elbows straighten. Bring your head up a little, relax, and repeat twice. Straighten up very slowly. This is a good stretching exercise for the back and the muscles of the legs. It also gives the neck a good stretch and lets fresh blood flow to your head. But, for that reason, you should not prolong the exercise by repeating it.

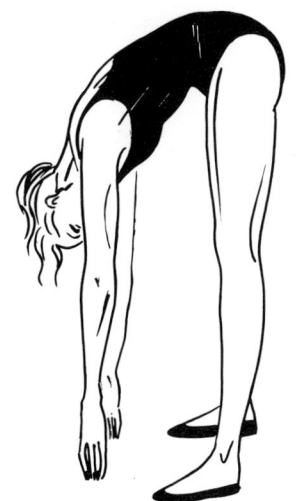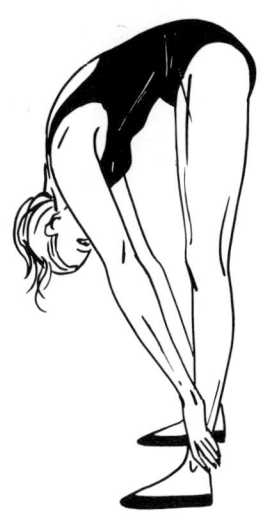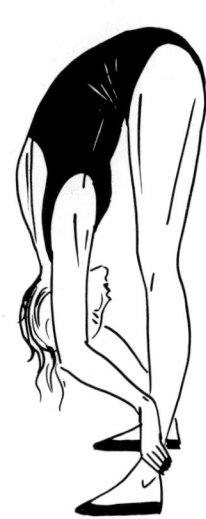

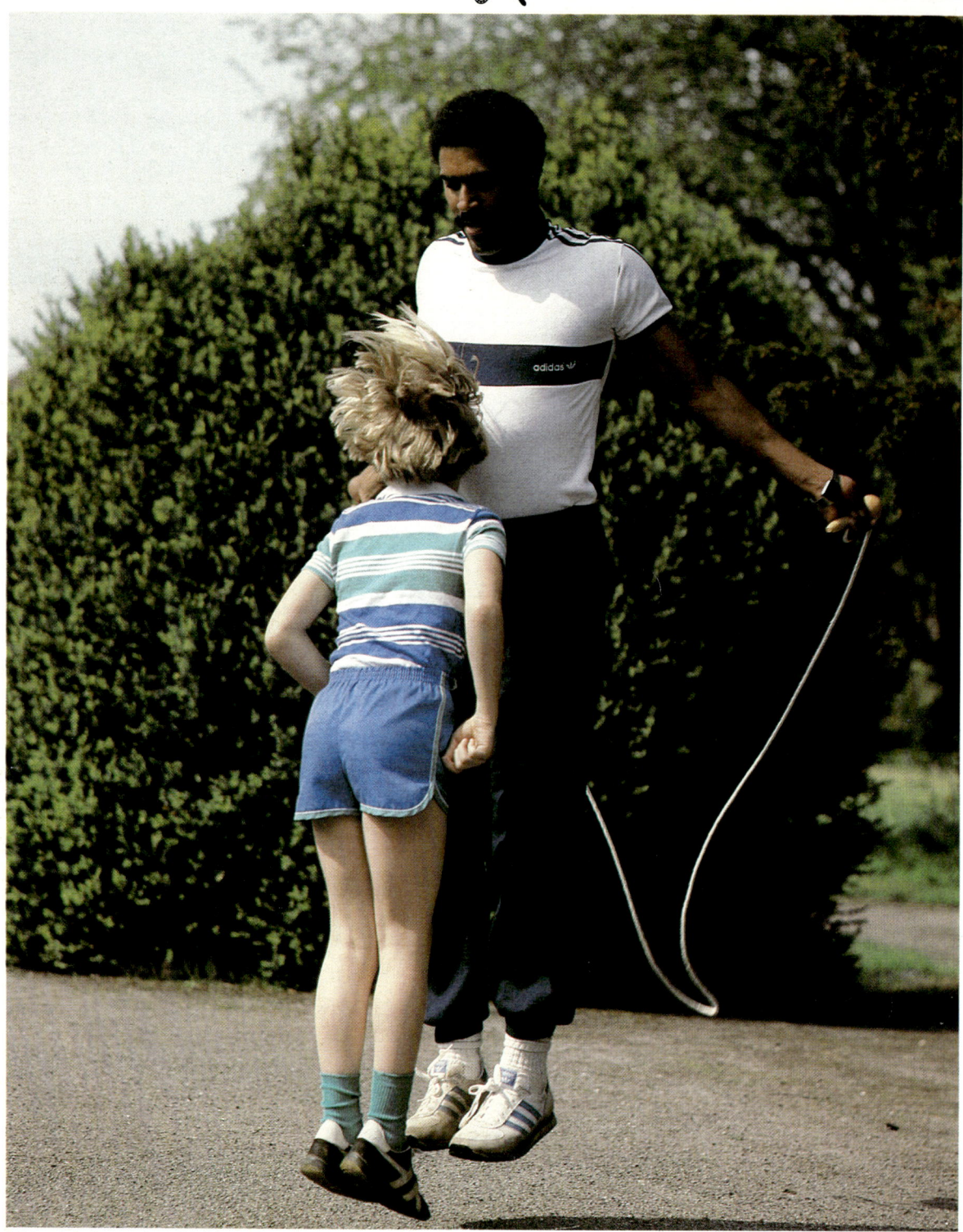

Skipping is not just kids' stuff! I thoroughly enjoy this excellent way of warming up and increasing general mobility.

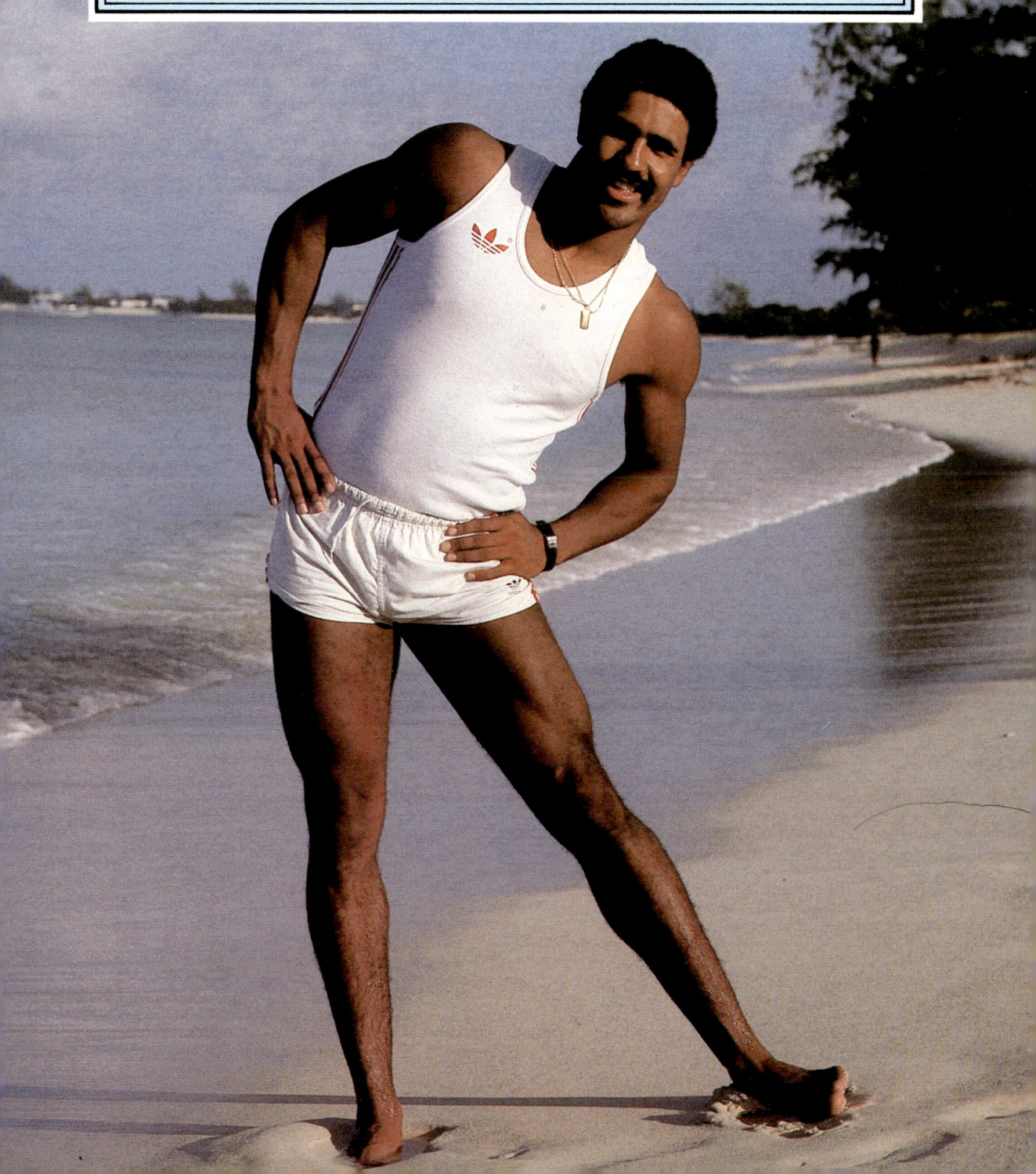

Chapter 4
Your Daley dozen

Get fitter in just twenty minutes a day, with my simple programme of twelve easy exercises. They have been worked out in consultation with my friend and fellow decathlete Snowy Brooks, who has used them successfully with people of all ages and stages of fitness at the London gym where he teaches. They have also been approved by sports doctors and athletics coaches.

When we decided to launch the programme, we aimed for twelve exercises which, between them, help condition every part of the body. If all twelve are repeated for the given number of times each day for a period of eight weeks, they will get you into much better shape.

You do not need any special equipment or even very much room for the programme. All the exercises can be performed on the living-room or bedroom floor in an average size home, or in the garden if you like. Try to have your exercise session at the same time each day – whether it is in the morning before you go to work, at lunchtime in place of a heavy meal, or in the evening. Make it part of your daily (sorry, Daley!) routine which is as natural to you as eating or sleeping.

What benefits can you expect? Well, the guinea pigs who tried the programme reported the following: increased energy, smaller waistlines, better posture, reduced tensions, better distribution of body fat, better sleep, more interest in sport (taking part instead of just watching!), increased zest for life and work! Side benefits also included more sexual interest, and more patience – which may or may not be connected!

The twelve exercises consist of four warming up movements, four slightly more strenuous movements, and four movements which give harder muscular work. There are two sets of exercises: for convenience, let us divide them between the fit and the unfit. I must warn you, however, that all the exercises are meant for physically sound people – if you have the slightest doubt about your health, you must check with your doctor before undertaking this or any other fitness programme.

Repetitions for both programmes should be five increasing to ten. Running on the spot: fifty paces for fit, twenty-five paces for unfit.

Study the step-by-step drawing of each exercise carefully before you start, checking that you know exactly how to perform each exercise. Do not strain yourself if the position will not come exactly right at first – just do your best.

If you are already fit, the exercises can form a very useful daily workout to keep you that way: they will ensure you get a top-to-toe workout every day. I have been using the programme myself in addition to my usual training as an easy morning warm-up at home.

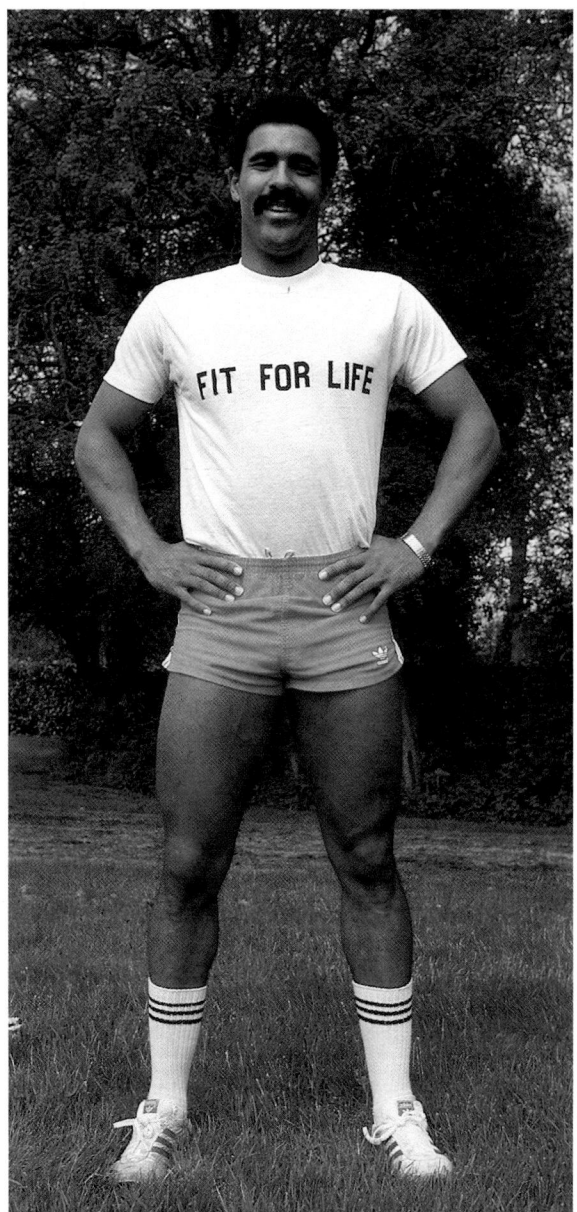

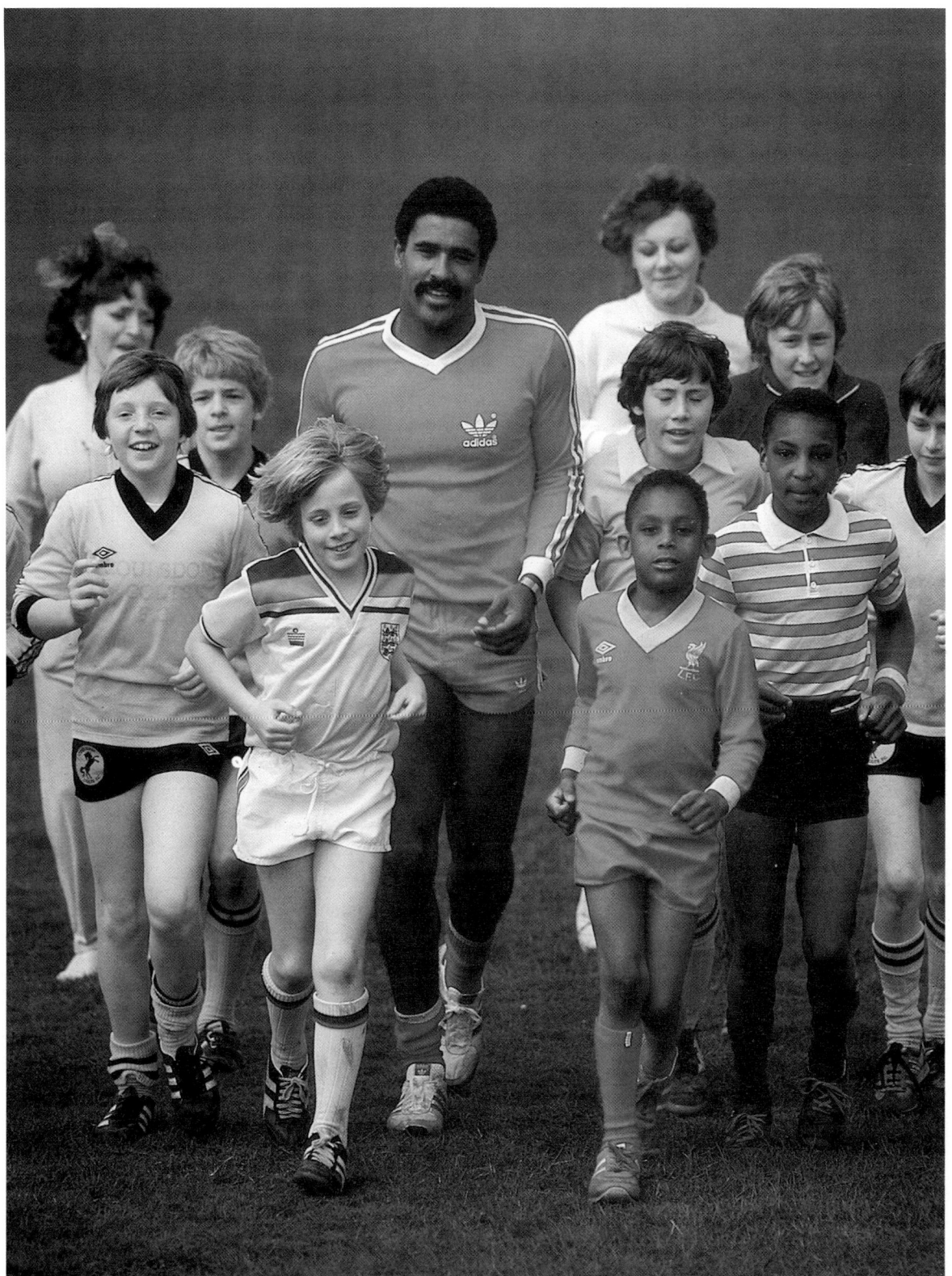

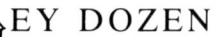

FOR THE FIT

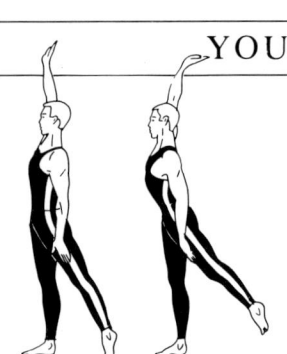

1 Leg and arm spine stretches

Stand straight, feet together, hands by your sides. Now take your left foot back, keeping your weight forward, left heel off the ground. Raise your right arm above your head. Raise your left leg and push your right arm back, keeping your right leg straight. Do set number of repetitions with left leg, right arm, then set number with right leg, left arm.

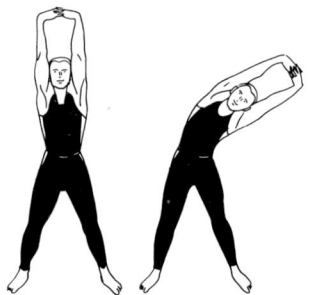

2 Straight arm side bends

Stand straight, feet about 90 cm (3') apart, hands by your sides. Now raise arms straight above your head and clasp hands, palms down. Move your torso and arms to one side as far as you can without moving your feet, or leaning forward. Return to starting position, then move to the other side.

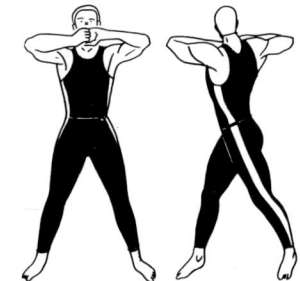

3 Trunk twists

Stand straight, feet about 90 cm (3') apart, hands up at shoulder level with fingers tightly clasped. Now, keeping your body straight, feet straight, raising the right heel, twist to the left as far as possible, to the front, then to the right.

4 Hamstring stretch twists

Sit on the floor, with left leg straight, right leg bent with your right foot behind you. Make sure your back is straight. Raise your arms to shoulder level

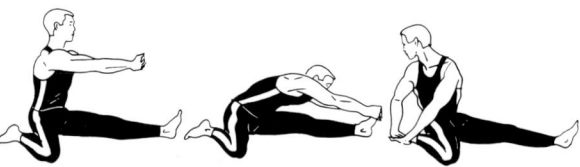

and clasp your fingers together. Lean forward slowly to try and touch your left foot (do not strain if you cannot quite manage it). Sit up straight, then twist your head and shoulders towards your right foot, aiming the palms of your hands to the ground, keeping your fingers together. Do set number of repetitions, then swap position so that the other leg is straight, and repeat, twisting to the other side, for the same number of repetitions.

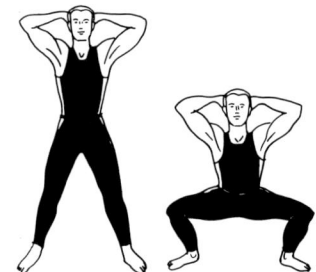

5 Squats

Stand with feet about 90 cm (3') apart, back straight, hands behind your head. Make sure your feet are facing slightly outwards. Now, keeping your back perfectly straight, squat down. Do not lean forwards – just go as far as you can. Straighten up slowly.

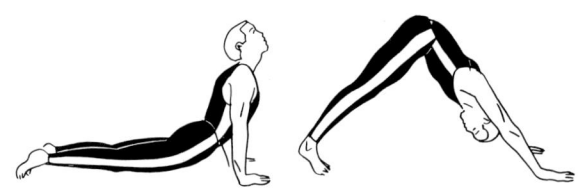

6 Back arches

Lie on the floor on your stomach, hands with palms flat on the floor at shoulder level. Straighten your arms and press down on your toes to raise your body slightly, keeping your back arched, head up. Push down with your hands, lift your bottom, straighten your back and try to push your heels back on to the floor.

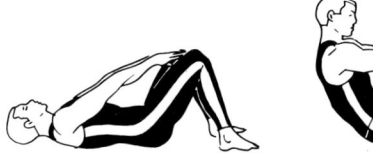

7 Bent knee sit-ups

Lie on your back on the floor, with feet on the floor, knees bent and legs slightly apart. Raise your arms to knee level, hands together, fingers straight. Leading with your head, roll up on your back to a sitting-up position, arms thrusting through your knees. Slowly, roll down, head going down last.

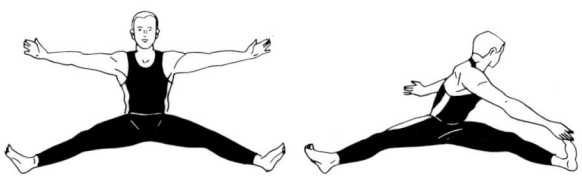

8 Wide leg twists

Sit on the floor, legs open as wide as possible, back straight, arms out horizontally. Keeping your arms and legs straight, turn the upper part of your body, head and arms to the left, so your hand touches your left foot. Do not bend knees to achieve this, if you cannot touch your toes, go as far as you can without straining. Straighten up and twist to the right.

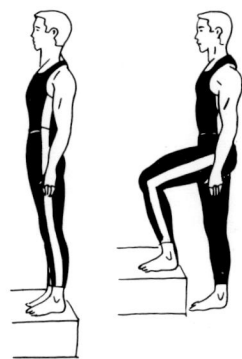

9 Step-ups

Stand facing a small bench or low chair or the bottom step of the stairs. Now step up on to the bench with your left foot, bring your right foot up to meet it, then step down with your right foot, bring your left foot down to meet it. Keep your back straight, hands by your sides throughout the exercise.

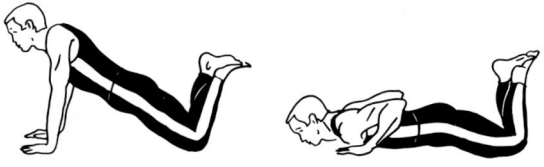

10 Bent knee press-ups

Kneel on the floor, place your hands flat on the floor in front of you, elbows straight, fingers pointing forwards, back straight. Now raise your feet, ankles crossed. Bend your elbows and lower your body slowly, so that your chin touches the ground in front of you. Straighten your arms, raising your body to starting position.

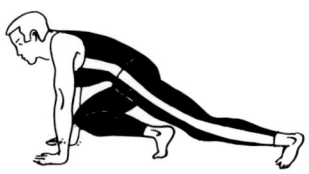

11 Single leg squat-thrusts

Stand straight, now crouch down, with hands on the floor, right knee bent, left leg straight out behind you. Now rapidly alternate legs in a running movement.

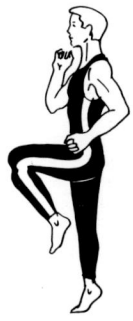

12 Running on the spot

Start with back straight, elbows bent. Now run on the spot for set number of steps.

FOR THE UNFIT

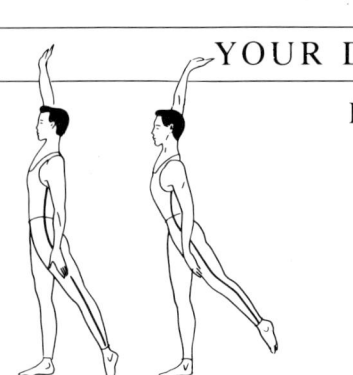

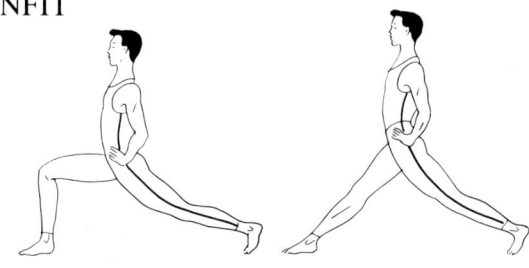

1 *Leg and arm spine stretches*

Stand straight, feet together, hands by your sides. Now step back with your left foot, keeping your weight forward, left heel off the ground. Raise your right arm above your head. Raise your left leg and push your right arm back, still keeping your right leg straight. Do set number of repetitions with left leg, right arm, then set number with right leg, left arm.

4 *Split lunges*

Stand with both feet on the floor, hands on your hips, with your right leg straight out in front, left leg straight out behind, legs wide apart. Now bend your right knee, moving the weight on to it. Keep your back straight and get as low as you can without leaning forward. Do set number of repetitions, then change legs and repeat.

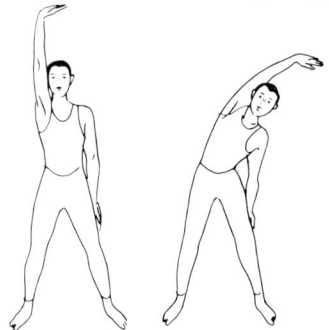

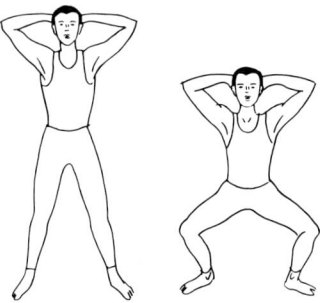

2 *Curved arm side bends*

Stand straight, feet about 60 cm (2′) apart, hands by your sides. Now raise your right arm above your head, and bend your body, from the waist only, over to the left as far as you can go. Straighten up and repeat to the right.

5 *Squats*

Stand with feet about 60 cm (2′) apart, back straight, hands behind your head. Make sure your feet are facing slightly outwards. Now, keeping your back perfectly straight, squat down. Do not lean forwards – just go as far as you can. Straighten up slowly.

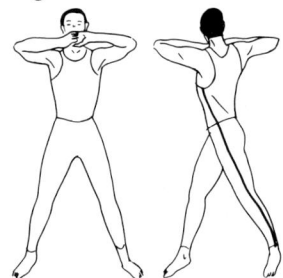

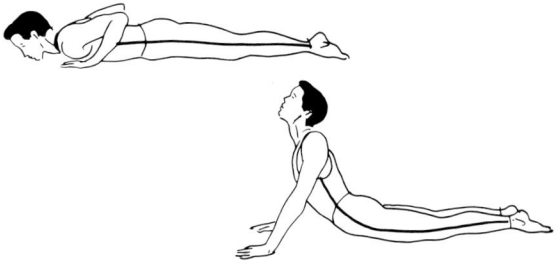

3 *Trunk twists*

Stand straight, feet about 90 cm (3′) apart, hands up at shoulder level with fingers tightly clasped. Now, keeping your body straight, feet straight, raising the right heel, twist to the left as far as possible, to the front, then to the right.

6 *Back arches for beginners*

Lie on the floor on your stomach, hands with palms flat on the floor at shoulder level. Straighten your arms to raise the top half of your body only off the floor. Look up at the ceiling, feeling your spine curve. Lower your body slowly.

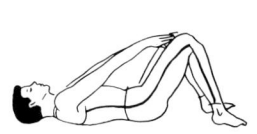 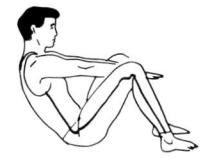

7 Bent knee sit-ups

Lie on your back on the floor, with feet on the floor, knees bent and legs slightly apart. Raise your arms to knee level, hands together, fingers straight. Leading with your head, roll up your back to a sitting position if possible, or go as far as you can with arms thrusting through your knees. Slowly, roll down, head going down last.

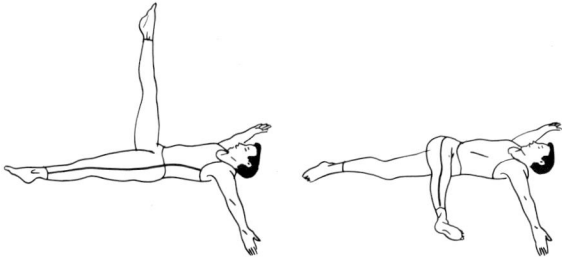

8 Straight leg crossovers

Lie flat on your back on the floor, arms out horizontally, palms down. Now raise your right leg as high as you can, keeping it straight. Flex the foot towards you and cross the leg over to touch the floor on your left as high as you can. You must keep your legs straight and try not to lift your shoulders off the floor. Repeat with the other leg. This makes one movement altogether.

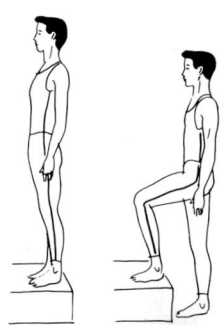

9 Step-ups

Stand facing a small bench or low chair or bottom step of the stairs. Now step up on to the bench with your left foot, bring your right foot up to meet it,

then step down with your right foot, bringing your left foot down to meet it. Keep your back straight, hands by your sides throughout the exercise.

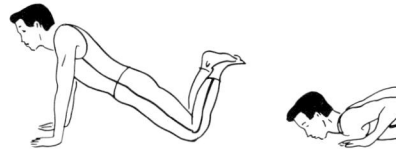

10 Bent knee press-ups

Kneel on the floor, place your hands flat on the floor in front of you, elbows straight, fingers pointing forwards, back straight. Now raise your feet, ankles crossed. Bend your elbows and lower your body slowly, so that your chin touches the ground in front of you. Straighten your arms, raising your body to starting position.

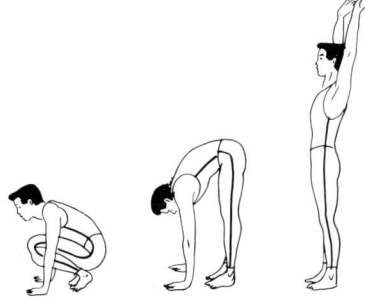

11 Squat, and stretch

Squat on the floor with bottom almost resting on your heels, hands flat on the floor just in front of your feet. Now straighten your legs, pushing your bottom into the air. Straighten up your whole body, stretching your arms right up above your head, swinging them down behind you. Return to starting position.

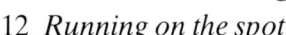

12 Running on the spot

Start with back straight, hands hanging loosely by your sides, or with elbows bent. Now run on the spot for the set number of steps.

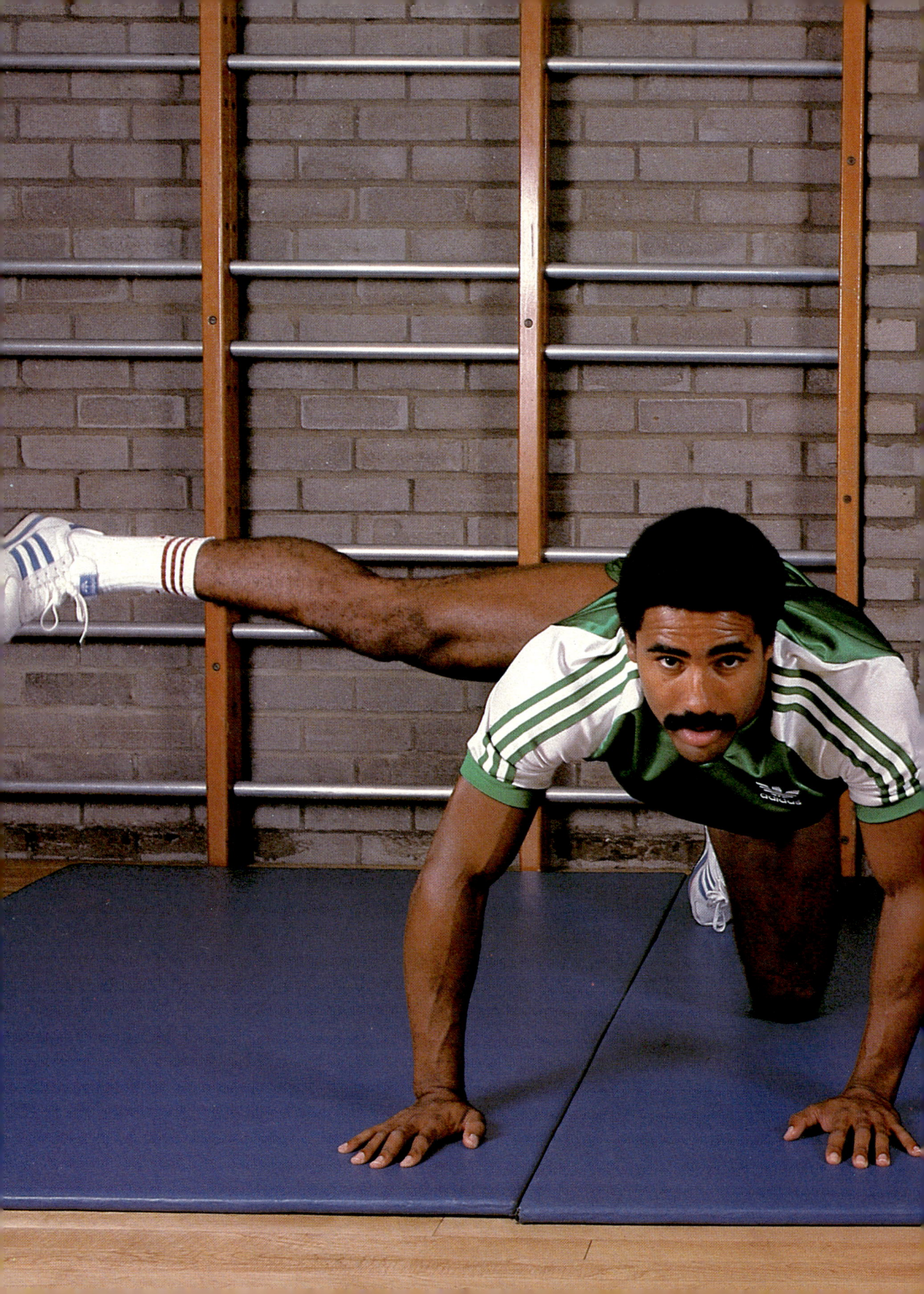

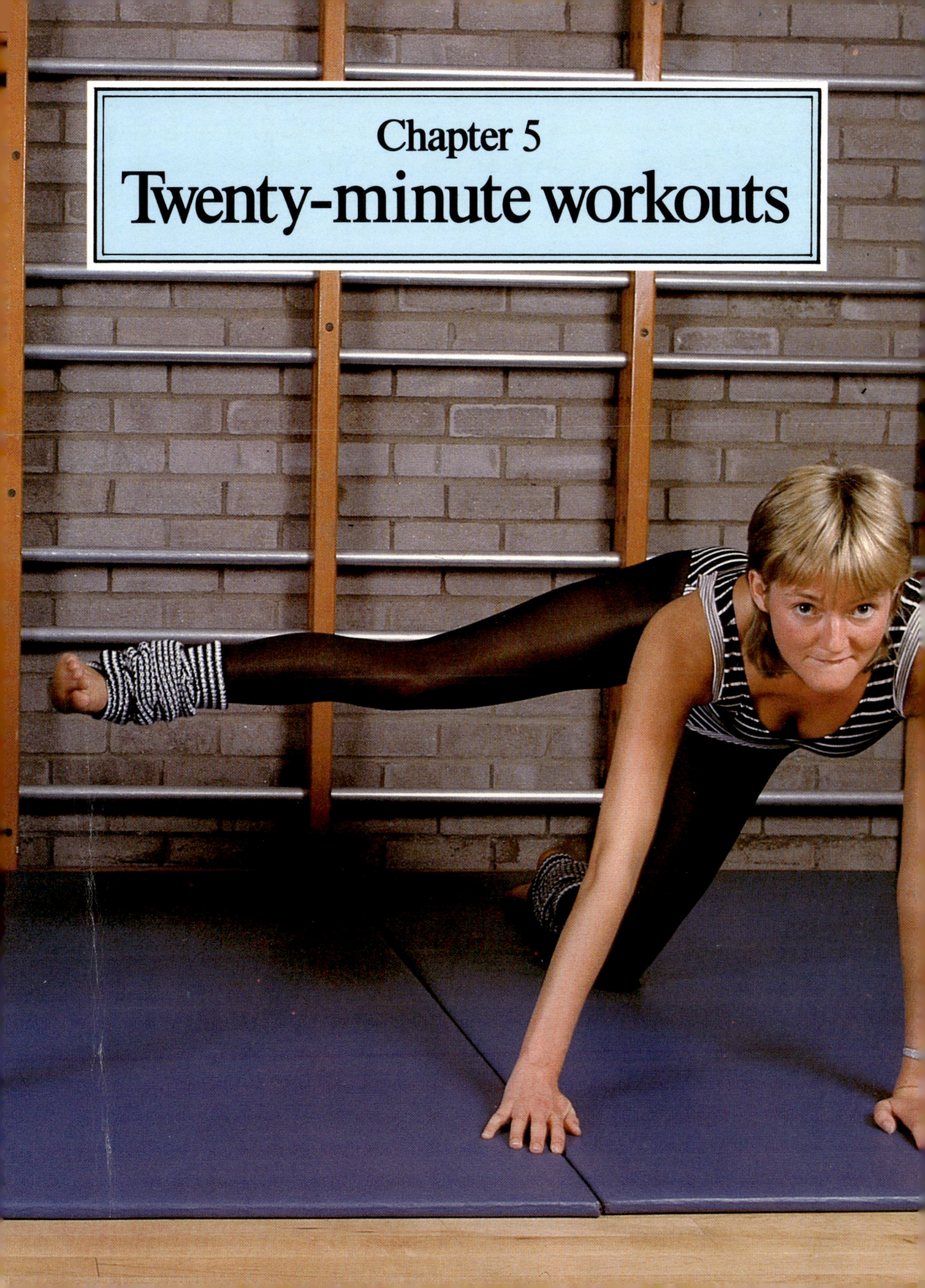

Chapter 5
Twenty-minute workouts

Here are four suggested workouts for people with different problems and requirements. Each one takes just twenty minutes, so that it can be fitted into even the tightest schedule. The workouts take into consideration the physical effects of certain types of job, plus age, and fitness level.

WORKOUT ONE

For the under-thirties in sedentary jobs

These exercises are lively, and fun, and concentrate on the areas of your body which are likely to need most attention after a day sitting down: thighs, buttocks, stomach, legs, spine, shoulders.

1 For spine, waist

Stand with feet wide apart, hands clasped above your head. Turn your body to the left, then lean forward from the waist, head down, arms straight out, keeping your head and arms in a straight line. Now circle the upper part of your body down, then up again, alternate ways. Repeat ten times.

2 For spine, stomach

Still standing with legs wide apart, lean forwards from the waist and thrust your hands through your legs, palms down, as far as they will go (do not strain). Now raise your body, place your hands on your waistline, and lean back. Repeat complete movement ten times.

3 For hips, legs

Stand facing a suitable solid piece of furniture, a chair or sofa-back, which should be at waist level. Place your hands on the furniture for balance. Now, keeping your heels on the ground, shoulders level, body upright, raise your left leg to the side, then swing down across your right leg and up again, as high as is comfortable. Repeat ten times, then ten times with your left leg. Now turn sideways on to the furniture, raise your outside leg up in front of your body, as far as possible, relax the leg and swing it down and back. Repeat ten times, then turn round and repeat ten times with the other leg.

4 For buttocks, hips, legs

Kneel down on the floor, placing your hands on the floor in front of you at shoulder level. Stretch your right leg out to one side, with the foot pointing forwards. Now raise the leg as high as you can, keeping it at right-angles to your body. Lower, repeat five times, then five times with the other leg.

5 For buttocks, hips, thighs

In the same starting position as 4, raise your left knee to the side as far as possible without straining, keeping your shoulders square. Lower, repeat five times, then five times with right knee.

6 For buttocks

Lie on your stomach, hands under your chin, feet together. Now raise your left leg as high as possible, lower, and raise your right leg. Repeat the whole movement ten times.

7 For release of tension in back, shoulders

Still lying on your stomach, hands flat on the floor under your shoulders, feet together. Now push down on your hands and raise the upper part of your body. Look at the ceiling. Repeat ten times.

8 For stomach

Lie on your back, feet together. Sit up slightly, supporting yourself on your elbows. Bend your knees and lift your feet up off the floor. Stretch out your legs and lower them to a point as near as possible to the ground without flopping. Bend knees again, raise feet, then lower them to that same point. Repeat ten times.

9 For legs, stamina

On your hands and knees on the floor, stretch out your right leg, leaving your left knee as high up to your chest as possible. Alternate right and left legs in a 'running' movement on the spot. Make ten 'paces' with each foot.

10

As you become fitter, repeat last three exercises three times.

11 For waist, relaxation

Stand with feet apart. Right hand above your head, left hand across your body. Now lean to the left in a

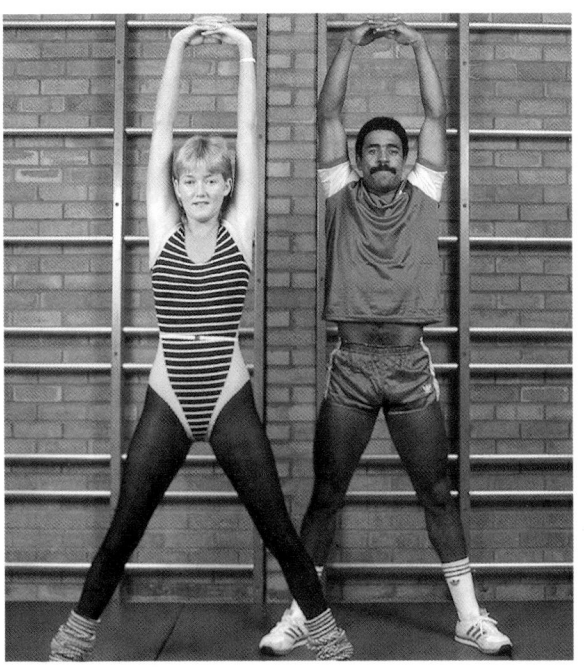

1a For spine, waist

relaxed movement. Bring your left hand up, right hand down, and lean to the right. Continue this rhythmic movement for a count of twenty.

WORKOUT TWO

For the over-thirties in sedentary jobs, and the under-thirties who are very unfit

These are very easy exercises and should be manageable for those who have neglected exercise for many months. They are also suitable for lively older people – but do check with your doctor before tackling them if you have back trouble, a heart condition, or are in any doubt about your health.

1 *For legs, general mobility*

Squat down on the floor with your bottom almost resting on your heels, hands flat on the floor just in front of your feet. Now bounce your knees and bottom up and down twice, and then straighten your legs, pushing your bottom into the air, hands flat on the floor. Never force the movement, just straighten until you feel a stretching sensation in the backs of your thighs. Now straighten up, stretching your arms right up above your head, and down behind you. Return to the starting position. Repeat five times.

2 *For hips, thighs*

Sit on the floor with your left leg straight out in front of you, right knee bent with your right foot resting against your left knee. Place both hands palms down on the floor behind you. Now roll your right knee over your left leg to touch the floor with the knee without moving your hands. Roll back so that your right knee touches the floor on the right. Repeat ten times, then change leg position and repeat with left knee.

3 *For legs, buttocks*

Stand at arms' distance from a wall, with palms flat against it. Now raise your right knee to your chest, then stretch the leg downwards and swing it up and backwards as high as you can, keeping it straight. Do not lean forwards. Repeat ten times, then swap legs and repeat a further ten times.

4 *For chest, bust*

Stand with feet apart, raise arms to shoulder height and bend your elbows so that your left fist is level with your right elbow and vice versa. Now move your elbows in and out so that your fists make rapid 'crossover' movements in front of your chest. Repeat thirty times, keeping those arms at shoulder height.

5 *For waist, midriff*

Stand with legs apart, hands behind your head, elbows out to the sides. Now bend your torso from left to right without twisting your body. Repeat ten times each side.

6 *For thighs*

Stand with both feet on the floor, hands on your hips, with your right leg straight out in front, left leg behind, legs wide apart. Distribute your weight evenly between your two feet. Now bend your right leg, moving your weight on to it. Keep your back straight, and go down as low as you can without bending forwards. Bend and straighten ten times, swap legs and repeat.

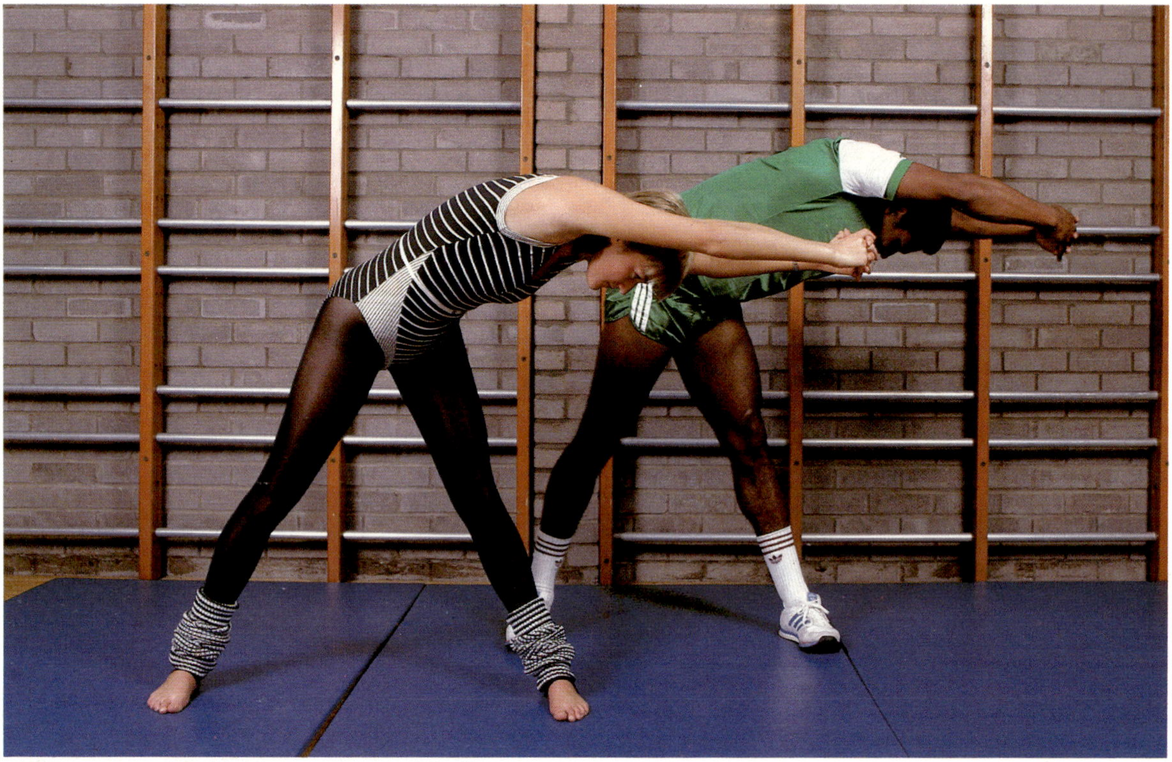

1b Keep your head and arms in a straight line

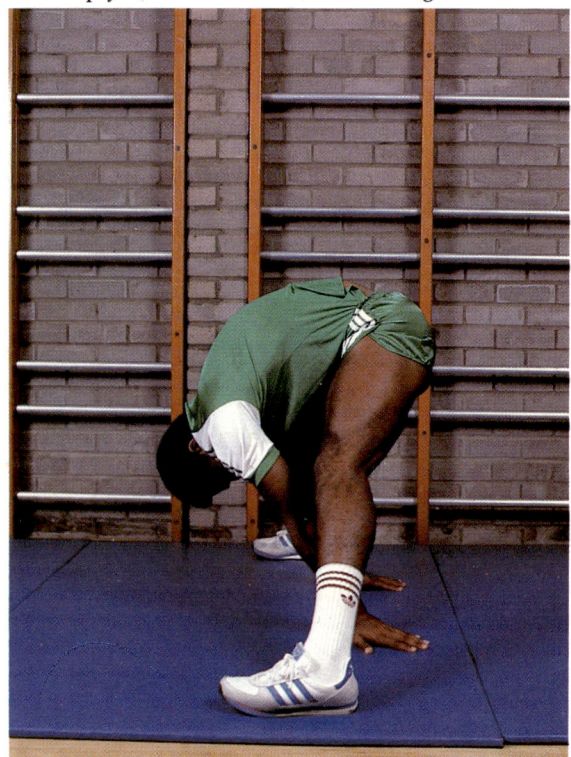

2a For spine, stomach

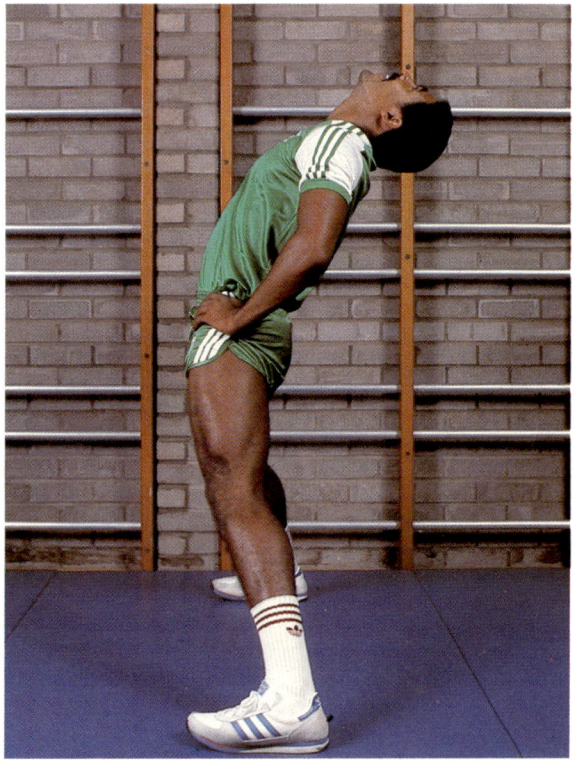

2b Hands on waist, lean back

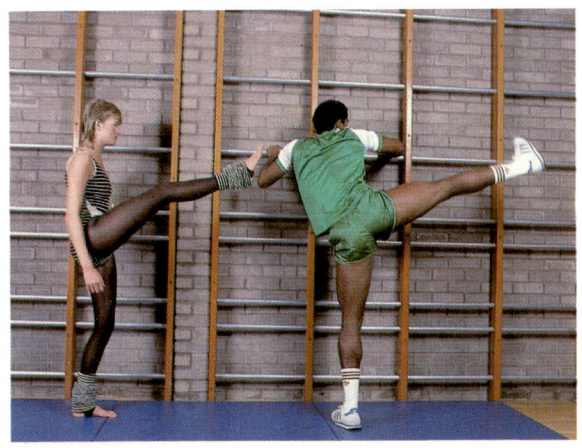

3 For hips, legs

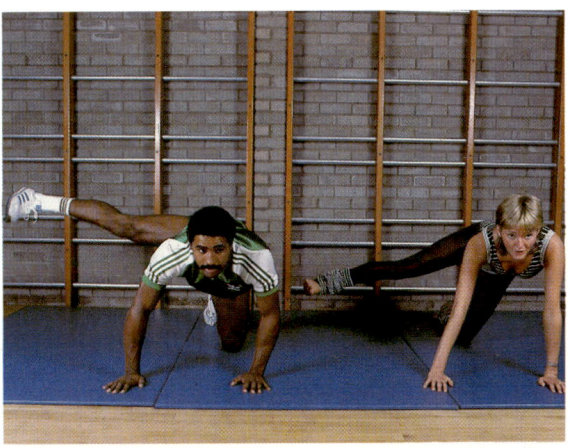

4 For buttocks, hips, legs

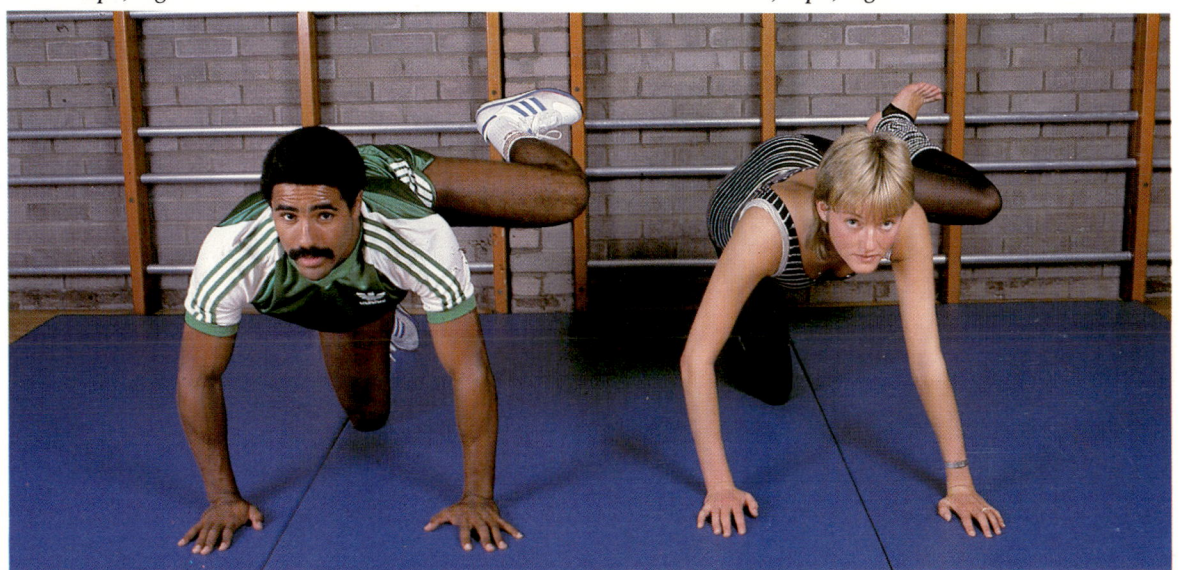

5 For buttocks, hips, thighs

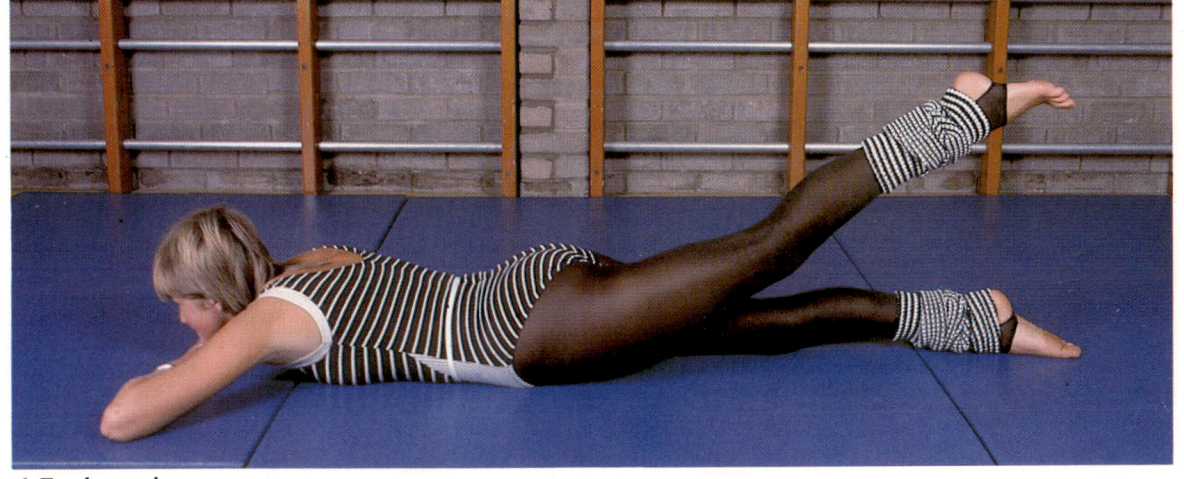

6 For buttocks

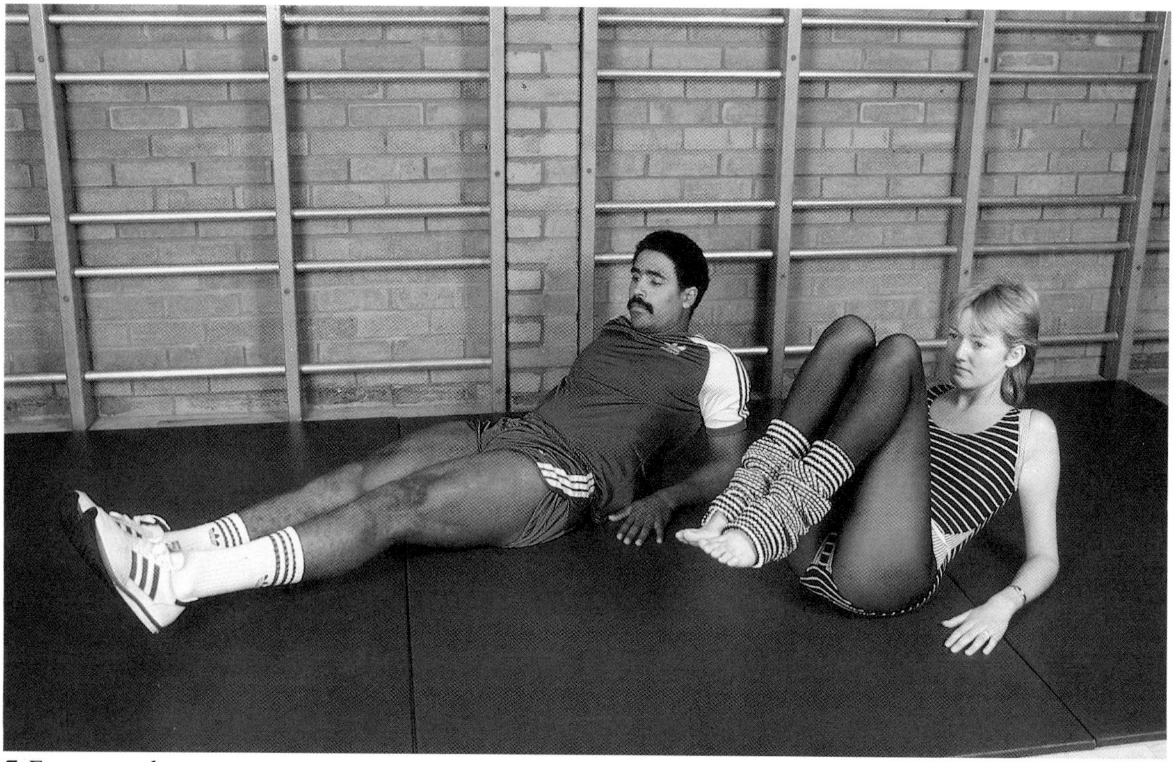

7 For stomach

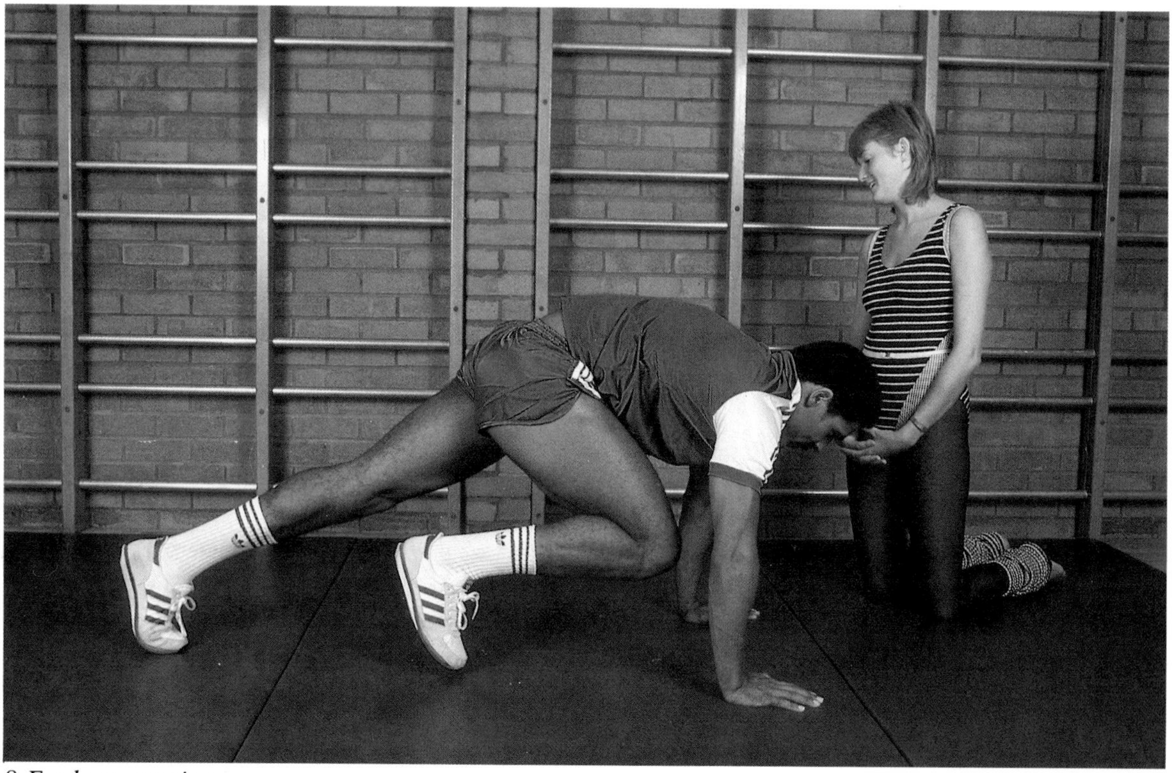

8 For legs, stamina

7 *For general stamina*

Run on the spot for a count of fifty, getting your knees up as high as possible.

8

Lie down on the floor and relax for five minutes.

WORKOUT THREE

For fit, lively teenagers and sporty adults

This routine will provide a good daily back-up to your general fitness campaign, helping you to maintain stamina and agility as well as muscle tone between sporting commitments. There is particular emphasis on arm strength, leg strength, stomach muscle tone.

1 *For warm-up*

Stand with feet apart, clasping a light weight (1 kg.) or object such as a large can of beans in both hands above your head with arms stretched up. Now swing your arms forwards and down between your legs, bending knees as you go (keep that back straight). Straighten your legs, swing your arms back up to the stretched-up position. Breathe in as you stretch, out as you 'curl'. Repeat rhythmically, as fast as you can, about twenty times.

2 *For chest, upper arm strength*

Stand with feet apart, hands by your sides, holding *two* light weights in your hands. Bring them slightly forwards, raise hands slightly, and bend and lift your elbows up and back, pushing hard. Lower and repeat thirty times.

3 *For waist, midriff*

Still holding the weights, stand with feet apart. Raise arms to shoulder level, and bend elbows. Punch right hand hard to the right, twisting round to the right with your torso (keep your hips facing the front), as far as you can. Return to first position and punch your right fist to the left, again twisting your body round as far as possible. Repeat twenty times.

4 *For stomach muscles*

Lie flat on the floor, hands by your sides, palms down, and feet together. Now raise both legs vertically. Lower your right leg almost to the floor, and, as you start to raise it, lower your left leg almost to the floor, so that the two legs cross in a 'scissor action'. Repeat ten to twenty times.

5 *For hips, legs, buttocks*

Lie on your back on the floor, arms out horizontally, palms down. Raise your left leg as high as you can, keeping it straight. Flex the foot towards you, cross the leg over to touch the floor on your right as high as you can (keep your shoulders on the floor and legs straight). Now repeat with your right leg, and repeat the whole movement ten times.

6 *For thighs, stamina*

Stand with your hands on your hips, right leg forwards and knee bent, left leg back with knee bent almost to touch the floor. Now jump into the air, crossing legs so that the right leg comes forwards, left leg goes back. Allow knees to bend on landing, then jump and cross legs over again. Repeat twenty times.

7 *For stamina*

Now run on the spot for a count of 100, knees up as high as possible.

8

Lie on the floor, relax and rest for one minute.

WORKOUT FOUR

For those in highly stressful jobs, new mothers, and those who work in cramped conditions
These exercises are all based on yoga movements, to help you unwind, stretch, relax.

1 *For neck, spine, buttocks*

Lie on your back, legs and feet together, arms by your sides, palms down. Bend your knees, raise your feet off the floor, toes pointed, and bring them in towards your chest. Lock your fingers, loop your hands over your knees, and pull them towards you, raising your head and shoulders off the ground. Hold the position for a count of five, then lower your head to the floor, relax for a few seconds, before unlooping your arms, and bringing your legs and arms back to first position. Repeat twice.

2 *For buttocks, thighs*

Roll over and lie on your stomach, hands by your sides, palms upwards, head on one side. Rest your cheek on the floor, let your heels drop open and relax. Breathe quietly and evenly for a few seconds. Now bring legs and feet together, place your chin on the floor, straighten your arms, make your hands into fists and push down hard, raising your legs off the ground at the same time, keeping knees straight and feet together. Hold the position for a count of two, lower slowly. Relax. Repeat twice.

3 *For neck tension, waist*

Stand with your legs and feet together, gripping your waist with your hands. Push your pelvis forwards a little, and bend over from the waist. Slowly roll the top half of your body around to your right, hold for a few seconds, then continue round to the back, allowing your head to go back a little (keep your shoulders down). Roll round to the left, and return to the front. Repeat rotation to the right, then relax from the waist down, and straighten up before repeating twice to the left.

4 *For back, legs*

Lie flat on your back, legs and feet together, hands by your sides with palms down. Now raise your legs, keeping your knees straight, feet together. Bring your legs up and over your head as far as they will comfortably go, pushing down with your hands to help the movement. Hold the position for a count of five, bend your knees in towards your chest, then slowly roll down, extending your legs smoothly. It is important to do this slowly, and with the minimum apparent effort, but it needs practice. Just do it once to begin with, working up to five, with a rest between each repeat.

5

Now lie flat on the floor, breathing evenly for five to ten minutes.

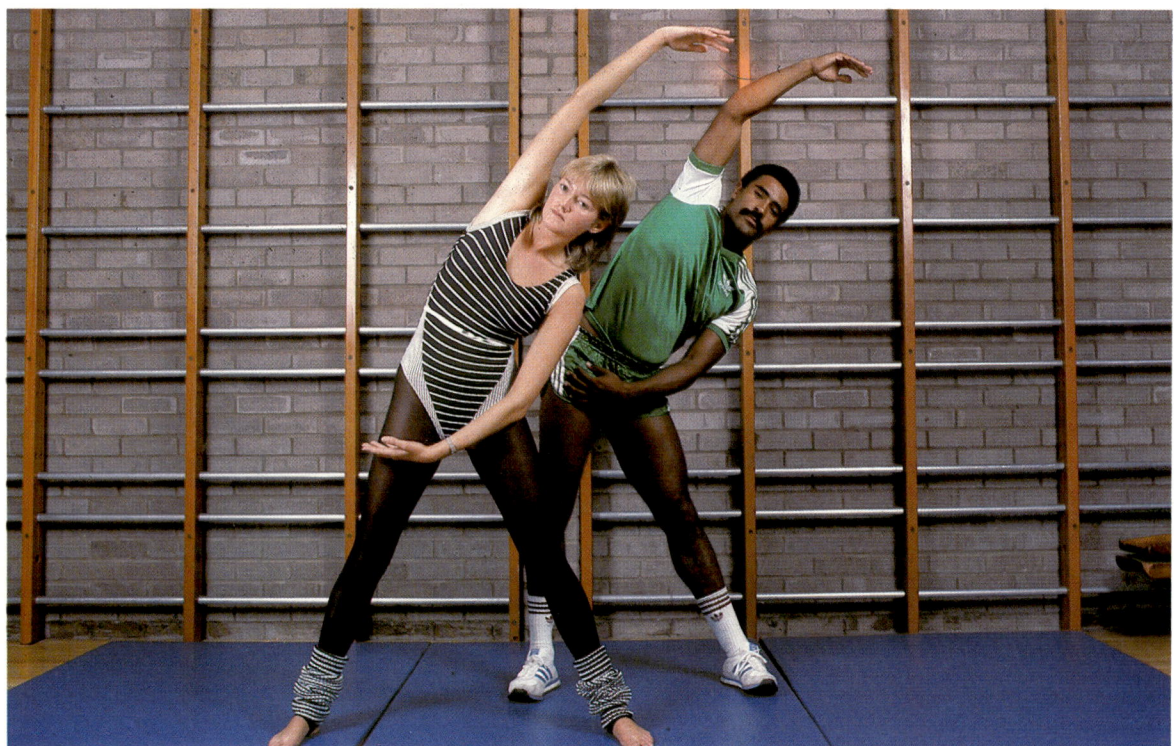

9 For waist, relaxation

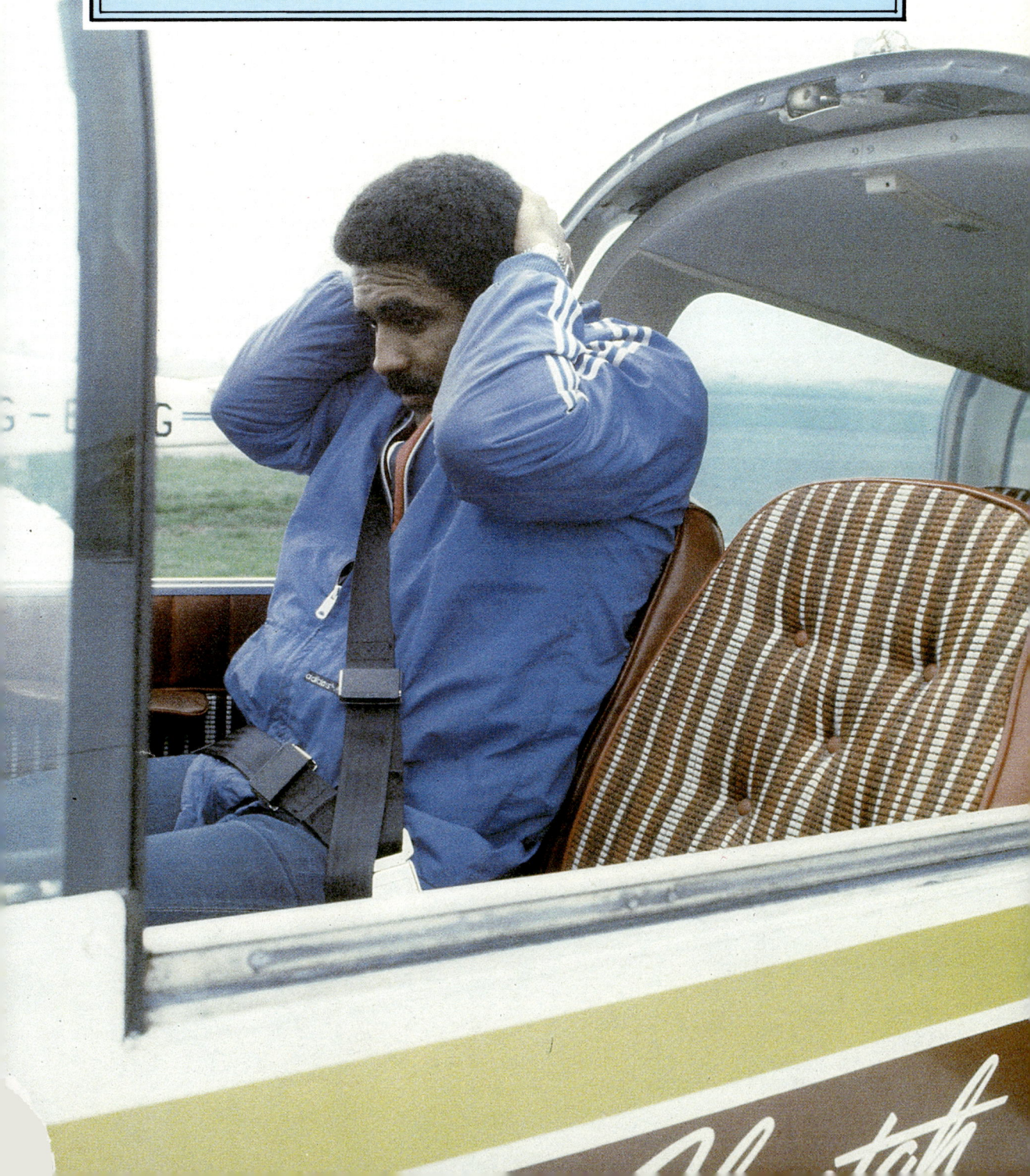

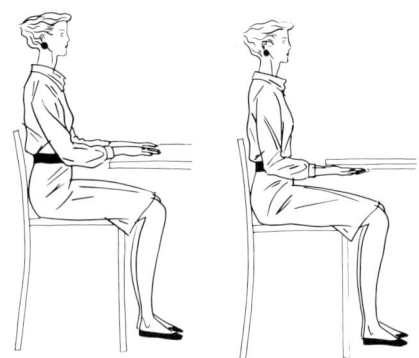

Athletes are frequently required to travel long distances by plane to take part in competitions. I hate wasting valuable training time sitting cooped up in a hot, sticky atmosphere – so I pass the time by doing isometric, or simple sitting, exercises, which take up little room but keep me feeling supple and relaxed. Of course, if the plane is half-empty or there are mainly other athletes on board, I shall be more energetic – using aisle space, seats and floor for a comprehensive workout. I do not advise this on a normal, scheduled flight unless the crew is very understanding! When I am travelling by train or driving for long distances, I also take the opportunity to do a few simple exercises. I recommend this for *anyone* confined to a small space – whether it is a train, plane, office, car, bath, or doctor's waiting room. If your movements are limited because of illness or handicap, this type of exercise is also a good idea. And it is ideal for people who insist that they have no time to exercise – for, with practice, such exercises become almost automatic.

ISOMETRICS

The principle of isometric exercises is simple: the muscle is contracted through pushing, pulling, squeezing or pressing against an immovable object. The force of resistance is brought in to act as pressure and the muscle is made to work very hard indeed, promoting strength, tone and endurance, without much huffing and puffing. Here are some exercises to try.

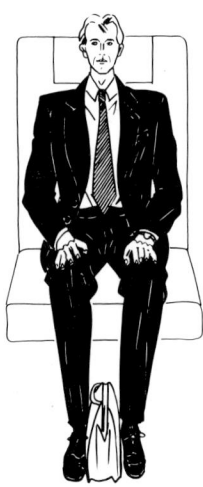

Exercise inside thigh muscles using briefcase

1 *For inside thigh muscles*

Sit comfortably, back straight, on any chair. Now find a suitable sturdy object – wastepaper basket if you are in the office, briefcase if you are on a plane – and place it between your feet. Squeeze your feet together as hard as possible for a count of six, then relax. You should feel the inside thigh muscles working hard. Repeat five times.

2 *For upper arms*

Sitting with back straight, feet together, place the palms of your hands on the table in front of you. Now press down as hard as you can, as if you were going to force the table down. Hold for a count of six. Relax. Now put your hands just under the table, palms up, elbows tucked in. Push upwards as hard as you can, hold for a count of six, then relax. Repeat each movement five times.

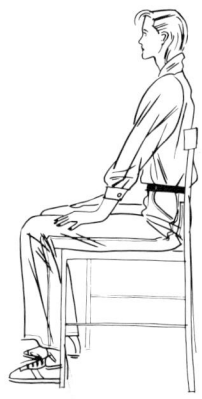

3 *For upper back and stomach muscles*

Sit with back straight, feet together. Now open your knees, and place your feet firmly on the floor about 30 cm (1′) apart. Place the palms of your hands flat on your thighs. Keeping your arms straight (this is important), press down, pulling in your stomach muscles at the same time. Hold for a count of six, then relax. Exhale *before* you pull in your stomach, inhale after the exercise. Repeat five times.

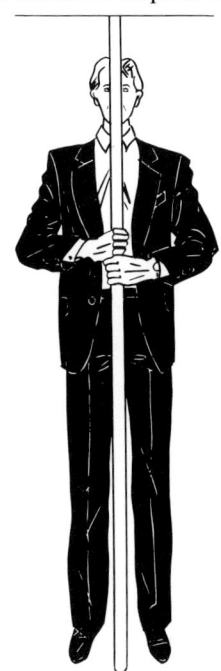

4 *For wrists and forearms*

Stand near a vertical pole of some kind (airport lounges are full of them, or use a bus stop or lamp standard) and grasp it with both hands, right hand above the left hand, arms bent. Now try to twist your hands in opposite directions, resisting the effort very strongly as you do so. Hold for a count of six, then relax.

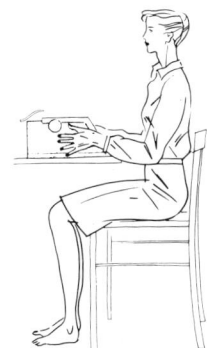

5 *For pectorals*

Sitting with back straight in your car or at your desk, grip the steering wheel at the nine o'clock and three o'clock positions, or place the palms of your hands flat against the sides of the typewriter. Now push

hard with elbows tucked in – you should see your bosom jump slightly if you are a lady – hold for a count of six, then relax. Repeat five times.

SIMPLE SITTING EXERCISES

These are very useful exercises for journeys – they are *not* isometrics, but use the normal muscle movement process. I recommend these (with your doctor's permission) for anyone confined to a chair by illness. They are also good for harassed sedentary workers who suffer from stress-related problems – often bodily tension is one of the main causes of stress, and these exercises can really help you relax.

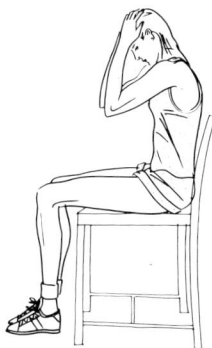

1 *For head, neck, chin*

Sit with your back straight, feet together. Now clasp your hands loosely around the upper part of the back of the skull, elbows forward. Relax your arms, pressing your head forward, chin in, until you feel a slight stretching sensation at the back of the neck (do not push, let the weight of your arms do the work). Hold the position until the tension stretching subsides, then relax.

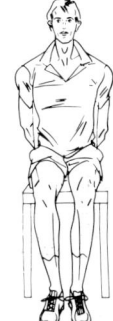

2 *For shoulders*

Sit with your back straight, hands clasped loosely behind you with elbows slightly bent. Now draw your shoulder blades together and push your upper arms together, without trying to straighten your elbows. Repeat three to six times.

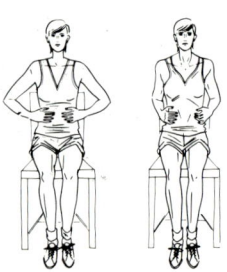

3 *For posture, shoulders*

Sit straight, feet together, with the palms of your hands on your lower ribcage just above your waistline. Now push your elbows and upper arms backwards towards your spine in sharp, short jerks – about six altogether. Relax.

Do not hunch your shoulders in any of the above three exercises.

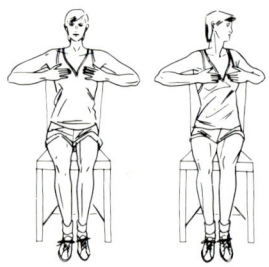

4 *For waist*

Sit with your back straight, palms of your hands on your upper chest. Now lift your breastbone and ribcage (which is likely to be drooping around your middle somewhere after a day in the office!) and twist your torso and head around to the left as far as you can, with your pelvis remaining static (legs relaxed, but *not* crossed). Now twist just a little bit more in short, sharp movements. Return to first position and twist to the right. Repeat five times each way.

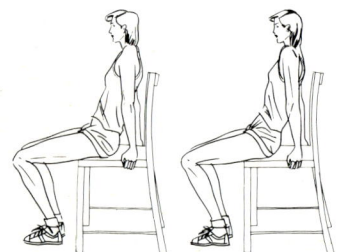

5 *For stomach and pelvis*

Sit near the front of your chair, with hands grasping the seat near the back. Now, keeping your back straight, lift your pelvis, so the pubic bone rises but your bottom stays put, in a rolling movement. The curve of your lower spine will straighten and your stomach will be compressed (you should exhale as you roll, to allow your stomach to be pulled well in). Relax. This is an effective but subtle stomach exercise and is particularly good for women who want to tighten up their abdominal muscles after having a baby, because the movement is gentle yet effective. Repeat five times.

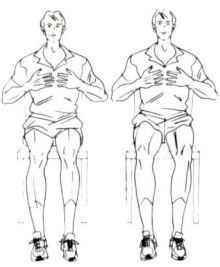

6 *For buttocks*

Sit with your back straight, feet slightly apart, and forward with knees slightly bent. Place the palms of your hands on your upper chest, contract thigh muscles and rotate them outwards slightly. Relax. Repeat both movements five times.

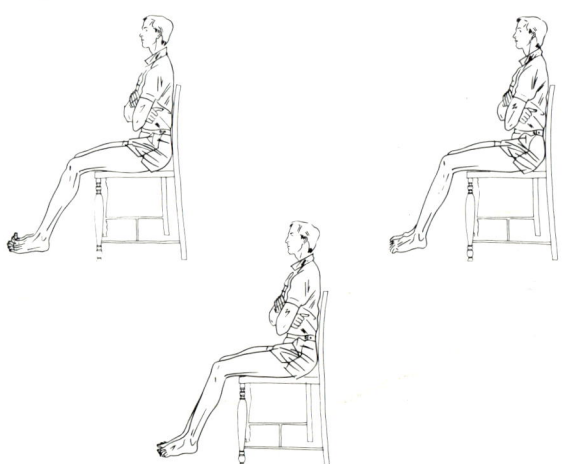

7 *For feet and ankles*

Sit with back straight, knees bent. Now bring your feet forwards slightly, heels together, knees together. Push your toes upwards and outwards, stroking them along the floor (this exercise needs bare or stockinged feet so that you can really *feel* what you are doing). Bring toes back together so that the big toes touch. Repeat five times, making sure that you try *not* to move your knees.

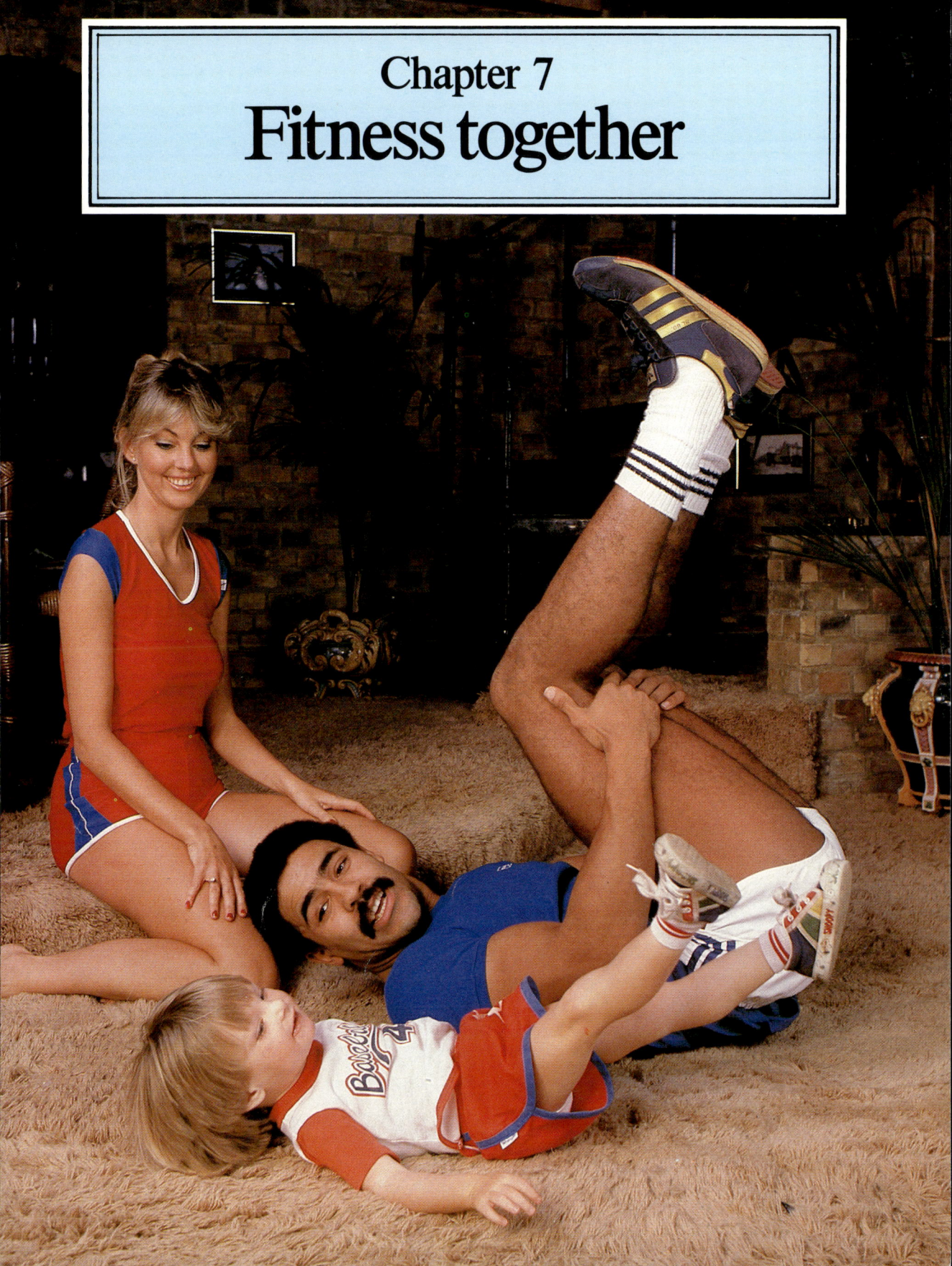

Chapter 7
Fitness together

Keeping fit need not be a solitary occupation – I am the first to admit that my friends, particularly the athletes I train with, are very largely responsible for keeping me on the straight and narrow as far as my own programme is concerned. Obviously, when it comes to the big build-up before an event, and the event itself, it is all down to *me*, and no one else – but I certainly do not enjoy too much isolation. Laughing at your own jokes is not a lot of fun! So, if you can enlist the help of a friend, or friends, you will probably find – like me – that keeping in shape is a real pleasure, even a social event.

PLAY-EXERCISES FOR MUMS AND TOTS

If you are at home all day with a young child it can be a break for you both to do some simple play-exercises. Children's developing bodies respond well to simple movements; exercise helps develop co-ordination, confidence, agility. It also gives a child a taste for exercise at a young age – encouraging an early interest in sports. If a child can learn that exercise is fun with mummy and daddy, he or she will be more likely to join in at school later on and really enjoy the fun. There is also evidence that a child who starts exercising early is less likely than a sedentary child to have obesity problems later on. Developing a taste for *action* could be one of the best early lessons you teach your child, though it is equally important to encourage him or her to *eat* properly (see chapter on nutrition p. 115).

Avoid any exercise which is too strenuous and keep repetitions to five or six at the maximum so that the child does not get bored. Have a set time for your exercise session – before lunch or tea, not after! – and slip into comfortable clothes so that the child can relax. Clear away any furniture first, and use a soft rug or carpet as your exercise 'mat'. You do not need very much space – the average sitting room is fine.

Here are six easy exercises which I have explained to a friend of mine, Gillian Duxbury, and her two-year-old son, Ryan. As a busy model and actress, Gillian found that her opportunity for exercising was restricted once she became a mum – there was simply no time to rush off to the health club or go to an exercise class. But Ryan, who is already a budding soccer star, was more than willing to join in this routine.

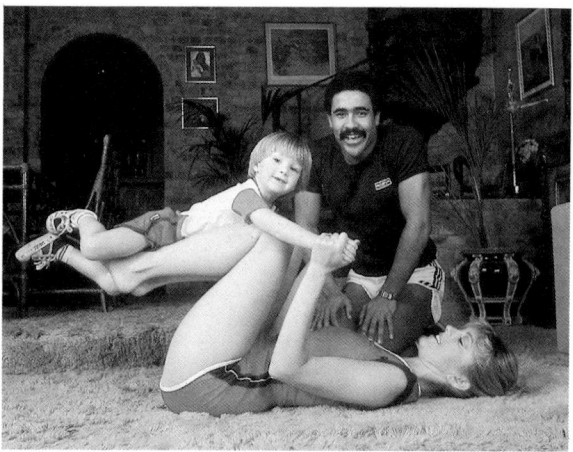

1 *For stomach, thighs*

Lie on your back on the carpet, hands by your sides. Now bend your knees up to your chest and raise your arms. Let your youngster climb on to your legs, stomach down, holding on to your hands for support. Now bend and straighten your knees slightly, giving the child a 'ride' down towards your stomach and up again. You must take all the strain on your stomach and thigh muscles, *not* your back. Repeat the movement five to ten times. **For you**: this will help tone up slack stomach muscles and inside and outside thighs. **For the child**: this helps develop a sense of balance and co-ordination between arms and legs – it is also great fun!

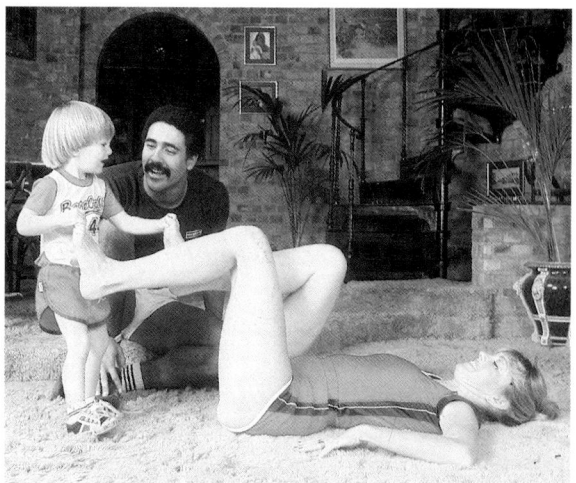

2 *For legs*

Lie on your back, arms above your head, and relax. Now raise your legs, and ask the child to grab a foot in each hand (no tickling) and push the left knee towards your stomach, then the right knee in a

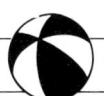
'steamroller' movement using plenty of strong action! Keep it up for a count of twenty. **For you**: this exercises the whole leg, and if you pull in your stomach while you are doing it, it also helps trim your stomach. **For the child**: a good movement for strengthening developing arms and legs and helping to exercise feet.

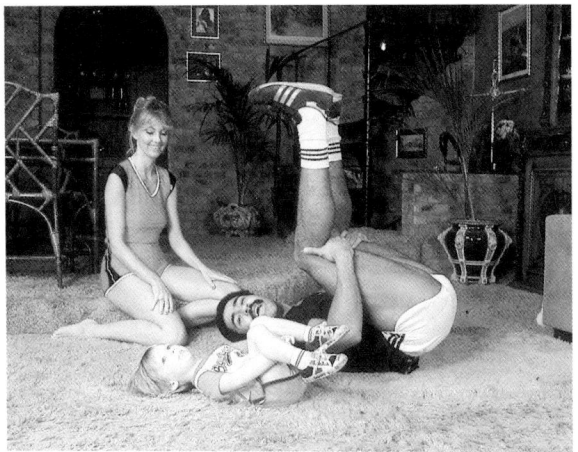

3 *For spine*

Lie on your back, grab the backs of your knees and curl your body forward. Now rock gently backwards and forwards, in a steady movement. Let the child do exactly the same thing. Keep going for a count of ten 'rocks', then stretch out and lie flat on your back. Stretch your arms above your head, your legs downwards, then press your spine into the carpet, almost feeling every vertebra. **For you**: the rocking movement helps keep your spine supple, is good for knotty shoulders, creaky backs and legs (I do this one every morning when I get out of bed to get my body going for the day). **For the child**: it helps keep the whole body supple.

4 *For arms, midriff, stomach, shoulders*

Sit back-to-back, a little way away from each other with knees bent. Hold a teddy or other toy in your lap. Now stretch up and back with both hands, still holding the teddy, and pass it backwards to the child, who should have his arms stretched up too. Lower your arms (both of you). Now it is the child's turn to pass the teddy to you. Repeat five times. **For you**: this is a great one for shoulders, especially if you have been hunched over an ironing board or stove. It also gives good muscle tone to arms, stretches midriff and encourages you to pull in your stomach. **For the child**: reaching upwards is a good

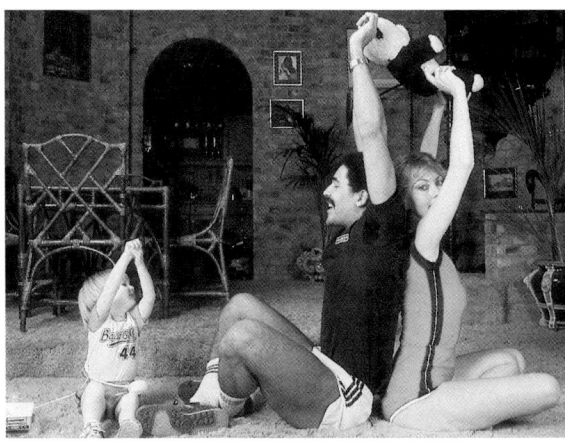

stretching routine for young bodies, and the 'passing backwards' exercise gives a dimension to co-ordination which is very different from the movements experienced during normal toy-play. The movement also helps develop a sense of balance.

5 *For back, bottom*

Go down on to your hands and knees, with hands pointing forwards, head up. Now arch your back, head down, and ask the child to walk or crawl through the 'tunnel' made by your body. As he walks back to his starting position, lower your back until it dips, head up, and clench your buttock muscles. Repeat slowly, with the child passing under the 'tunnel' five times. **For you**: this eases back strain, and helps to trim your bottom. **For the child**: this gives good, natural movement to arms, legs, the whole body.

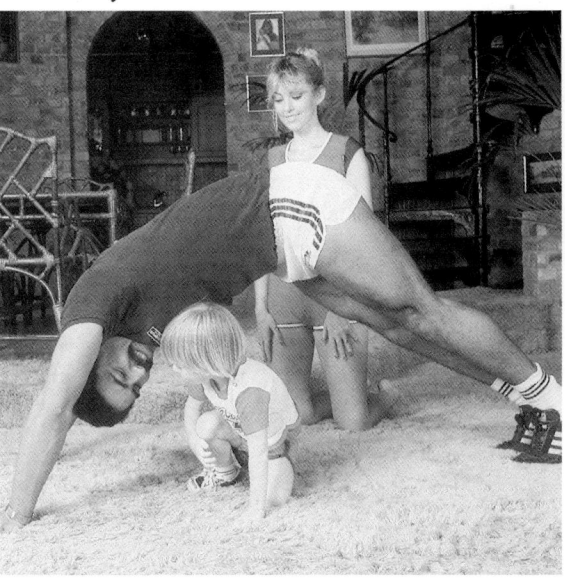

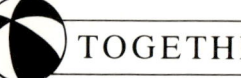

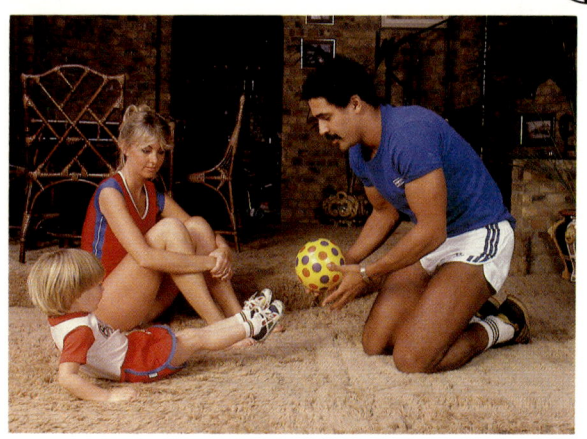

6 *For stomach, legs*

Get the child to lie on his back, raising himself up on his forearms. Now throw a ball for him to kick back to you ten times. Repeat, this time lying on your back yourself. **For you**: this is good for stomach muscles and legs. **For the child**: this helps develop a sense of co-ordination.

OH BABY – WHAT A BODY!

Perhaps the most important 'twosome' of all is a pregnant mum and her unborn baby. There is no need to stop exercising when you become pregnant – in fact, it is extremely important to keep your body fit and supple for the big day. Ante-natal classes will give you instruction in the vital breathing techniques and relaxation necessary for an easy labour and birth, and it is a good idea to practise these at home every day.

During pregnancy, your skin obviously stretches to accommodate the baby – but actual ligaments and joints loosen too. You need to make sure your body is supple during pregnancy to avoid aches and creaks – especially in your leg muscles, which have to carry that extra 10 kg (22 lb), or so, of additional weight. If these muscles are strong and supple (walk as much as you can – with your doctor's permission), you will avoid cramps, varicose veins and tiredness. Good posture is very important, too; the natural thing to do is to lean back as your stomach expands, but you should make a real effort to stand up straight (the right shoes are vital – not *too* high) in order to avoid backache.

Nowadays, many mothers choose to have their babies in a squatting, rather than lying down, position, feeling that this is a more natural way for the human animal to reproduce. Having watched some of the fascinating television programmes on this subject, I tend to agree. But do not forget that these days the human animal has become a bit rusty about *walking* – so many women have rather weak thigh and calf muscles, and hip joints, which are all vitally important during a squatting or standing birth. So, you really should prepare your body for the happy event, which is far more earth-shattering than any mere athletics competition – although a lot less painful!

Here is a group of good, gentle exercises for mums-to-be, and which would be equally good for anyone needing a non-strenuous routine after an illness or a prolonged period of inactivity:

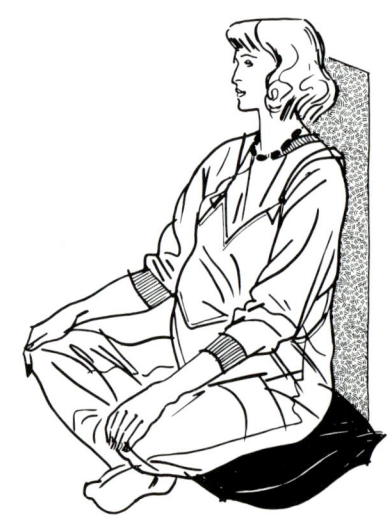

1 *For spine, hips, knees, feet*

Sit on a cushion on the floor, legs crossed at the ankles,* with your back against a wall. Now breathe in and straighten your spine, feeling each vertebra against the wall and lifting your front ribs. Relax and repeat. Stand up slowly afterwards.

*Although it is necessary to cross your ankles for this exercise, you should avoid constricting blood-flow by crossing your legs when sitting down at work or watching TV. Always sit in an upright chair, as it is much more comfortable than slouching on a sofa.

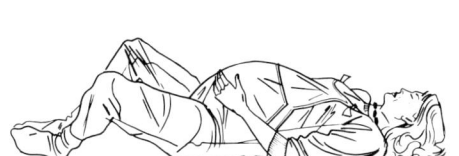

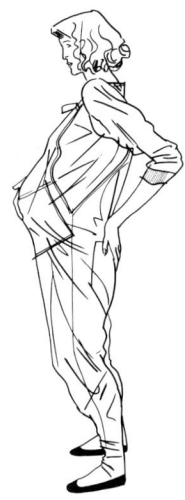

2 *For hips, knees, legs, feet*

Lie on your back on the carpet, arms loosely relaxed, hands on your stomach. Now place the *soles* of your feet together, let your knees fall outwards and pull in your stomach muscles. Hold briefly, then relax. Repeat five times.

Note: always roll over on to your *side* before getting up from the lying down exercises.

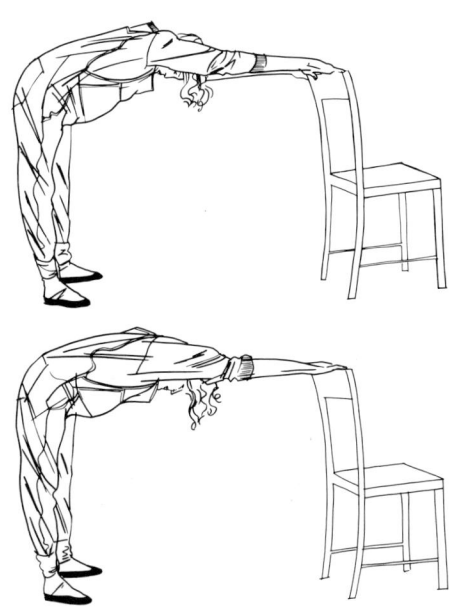

4 *For posture*

Stand with your feet apart, knees slightly bent. Now place one hand on your 'bump', the other on your bottom – just above cheek-level! Make sure your fingers point downwards. Now breathe in slowly and, as you breathe out, tilt your pelvis, lifting your pubic bone forwards and upwards. Hold position for a count of five (breathe normally), tightening up your pelvic floor muscles at the same time. Relax.

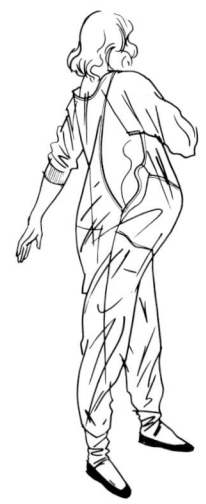

3 *For back, legs*

Stand, arms' distance from a chair or sofa-back so that it will be at about shoulder-height. Now, with feet slightly apart, bend forwards from your hips and stretch your arms out, resting your hands on the chair-back. Straighten your spine (feel that tension easing between your shoulders?), pull in your stomach and push down very slightly – do not strain. Stand up slowly and repeat once. You must keep your legs straight throughout the exercise.

5 *For spine*

Stand with feet slightly apart, back straight, in front of a mirror if possible. Your feet stay put as you twist your body very gently to the left, then the right. Repeat five times.

Check all exercise routines through with your doctor or midwife first.

A MINI WORKOUT FOR TWO

Here are some easy exercises for two fit, lively youngsters. Try them as a fun, mini workout on Saturday mornings, or after school. They will help build good team-work, as well as muscular strength and co-ordination.

1 For stomach, hamstrings

One partner should lie on the floor, arms overhead, and the other stand just in front of his feet, facing his head. Now the lying partner should lift his feet and place them at the standing partner's waist. The lying partner must fling his arms forwards and up, raising the upper part of his body to try and touch his partner's shoulders. Repeat five times, then swap over and repeat a further five times.

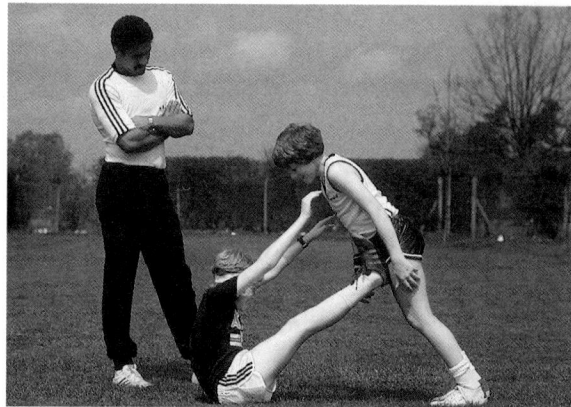

1 For stomach, hamstrings

2 For hamstrings and lower back flexibility

Sit opposite each other, legs widespread, with feet braced against each other's feet. (If one partner is slightly shorter, he should rest his feet against his partner's calves.) Now hold hands, backs straight. Slowly, one partner should lean back, exerting a steady, non-jerky pull, while the other one leans forwards letting his muscles and torso relax. Repeat the see-saw movement ten times.

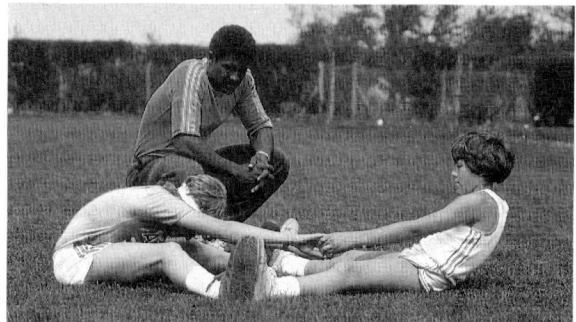

2 For hamstrings, back flexibility

3 For stronger thigh muscles, heels

Stand facing each other, holding hands, feet shoulders' distance apart. Now, keeping your back straight, do a full knees bend. Try to keep your heels on the ground. Straighten up, and repeat five times.

4 For legs, arms, back strength

Stand back to back, a few feet apart. Link arms, and place feet slightly apart for good balance. Now press your backs together, and go down slowly into a full knees bend, then return to standing position. Repeat four times.

5 For a stronger stomach, a slim, firm waist

One partner should lie on the floor, knees bent with feet fairly wide apart, hands clasped behind his head. The other should kneel in front and press both ankles as an 'anchor'. The lying partner should roll over on to the right shoulder and lift his upper body towards the sit-up position, leading with the left elbow towards the right knee. Touch the knee if you can, if not go as far as possible, then lower your body

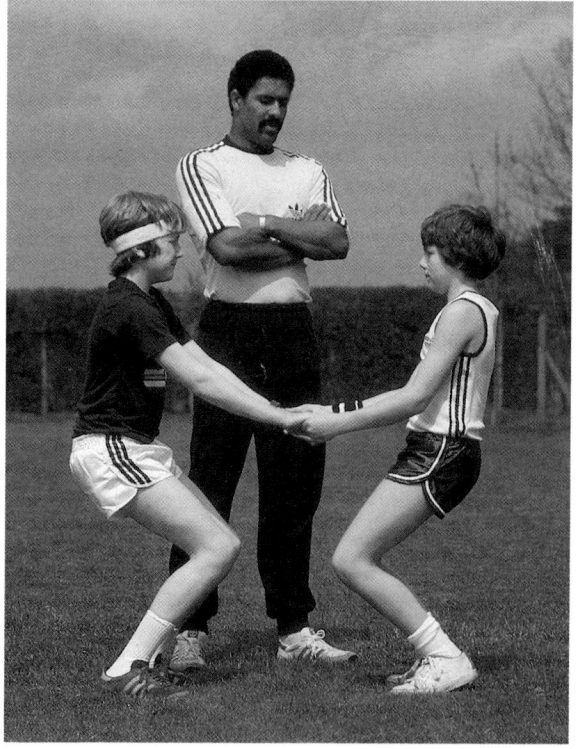

3a For stronger thigh muscles, heels

gently (do not flop). Repeat with right elbow, left knee. Repeat the whole exercise five times.

6 *For leg muscles, feet, and foot co-ordination*

Stand facing each other, holding hands, backs straight. Now 'scissor' both feet past each other for a count of twenty.

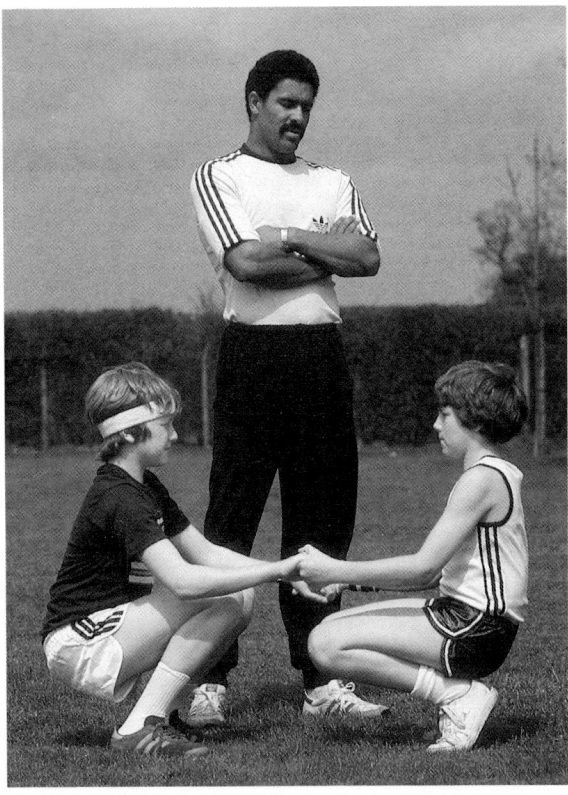

3b Try to keep those heels on the ground!

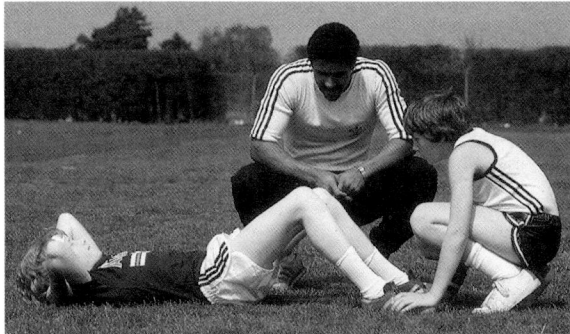

5a For strong stomach, firm waist

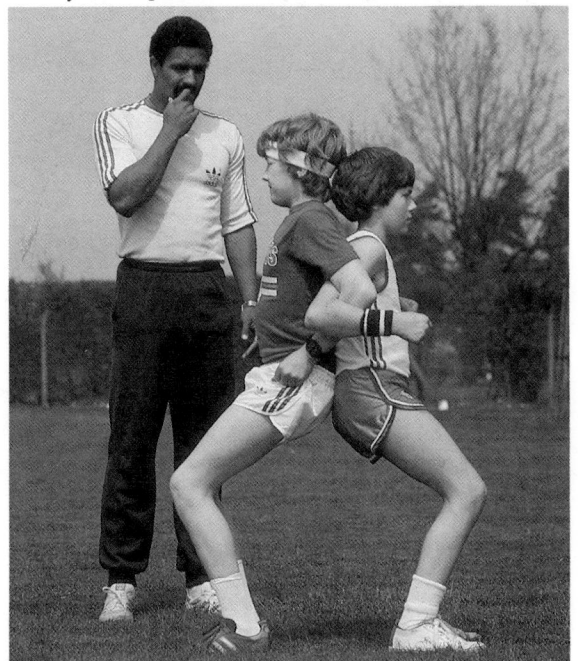

4 For legs, arms, back strength

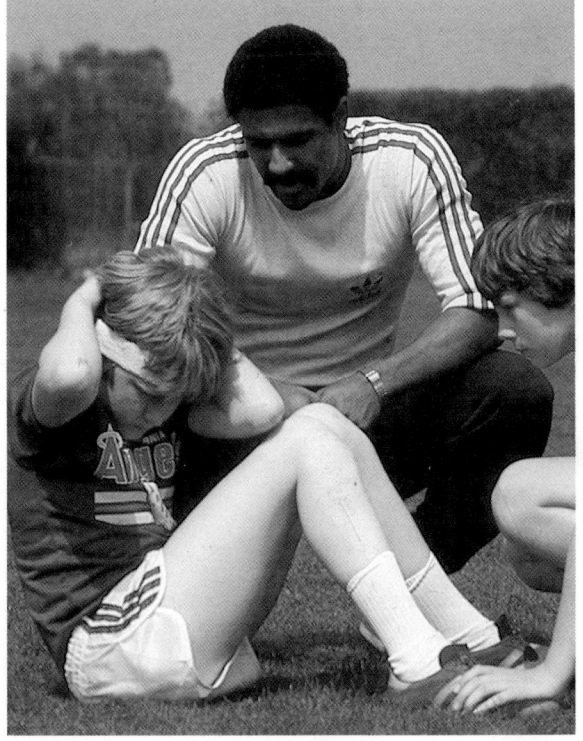

5b Touch your right knee with your left elbow!

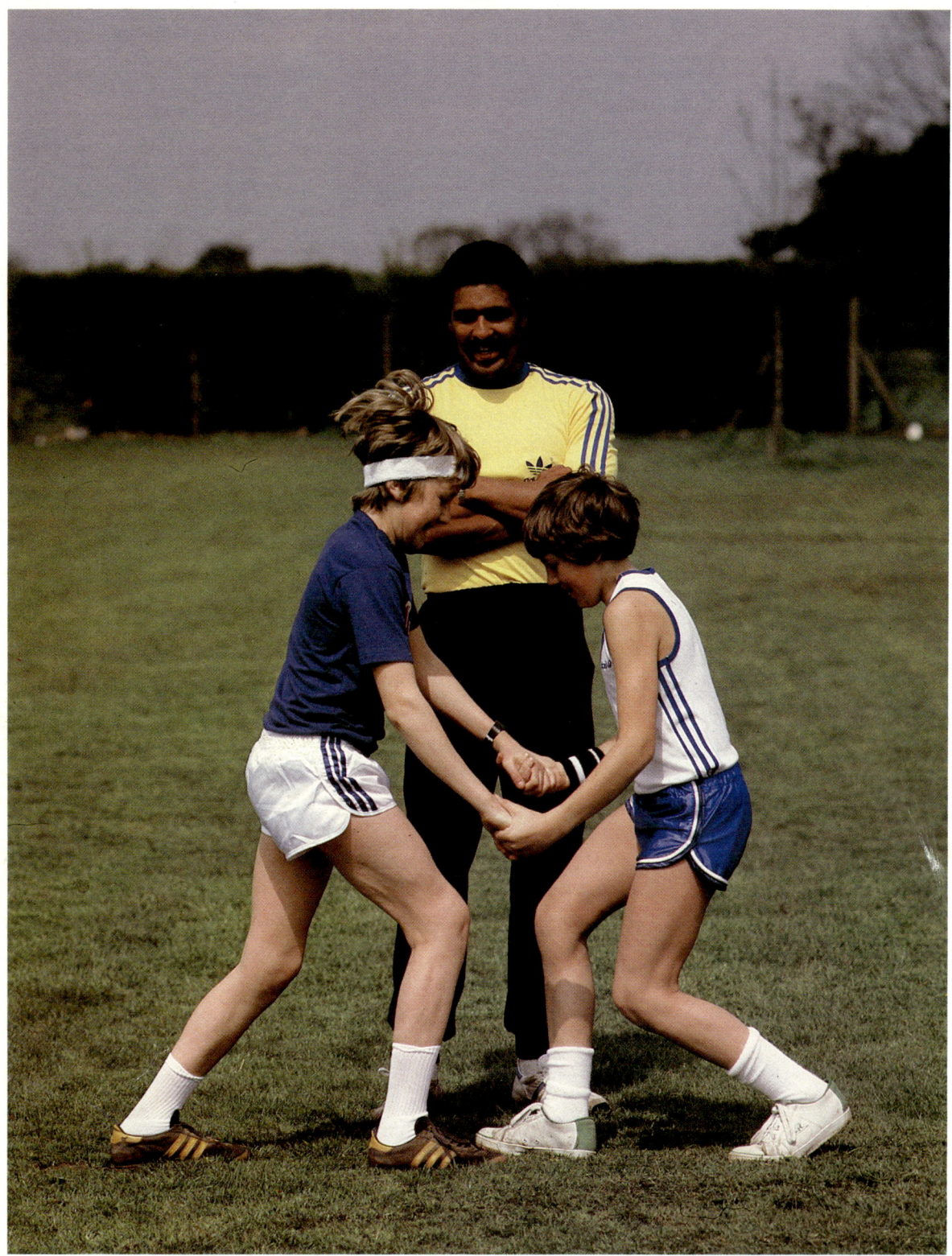

6 *For leg muscles, feet, and foot co-ordination*

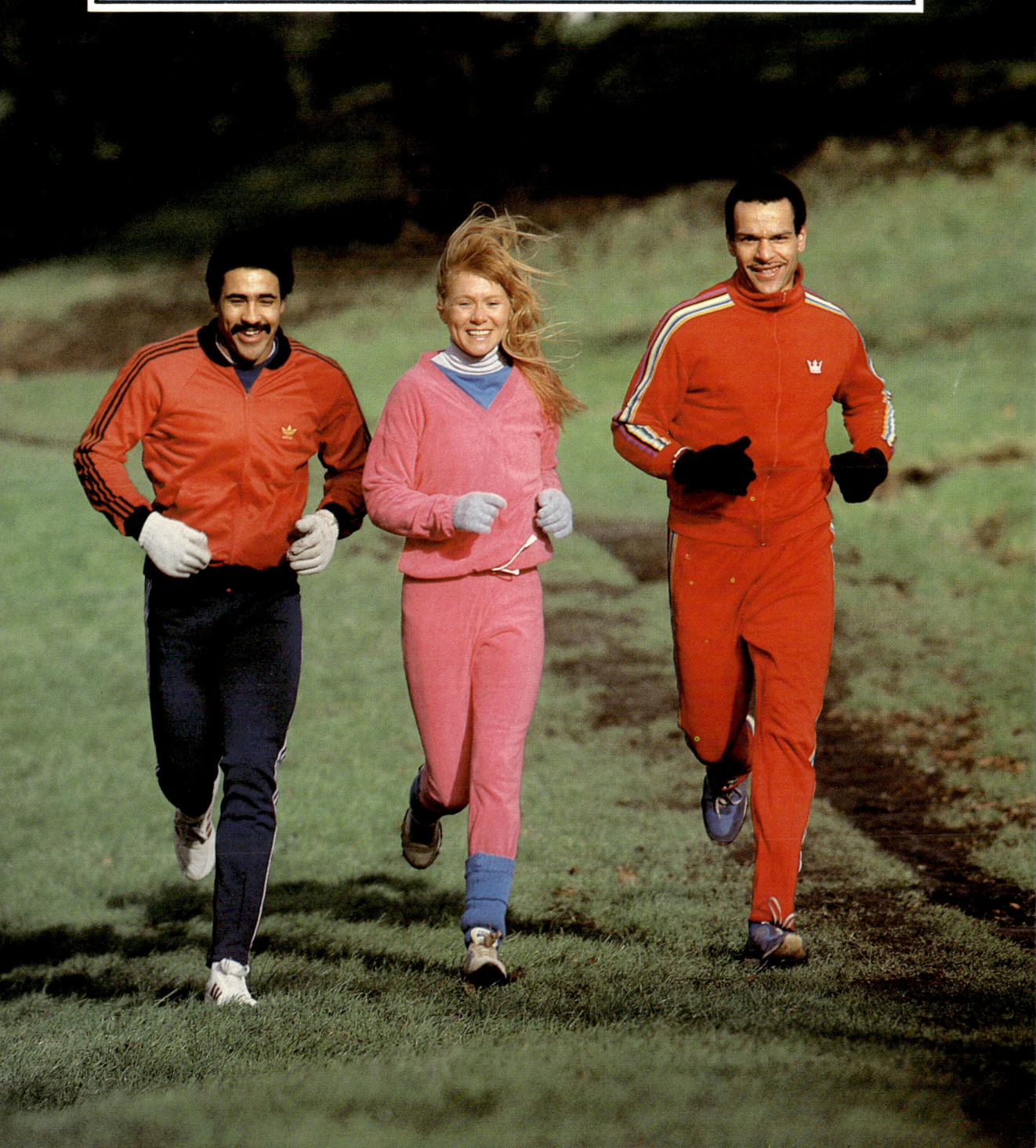

Chapter 8
Run for it

Whether you are a budding athlete, footballer, dancer or squash-player – or just a sedentary worker who wants to stay trim – running can be a fun way to keep fit. When I say 'fun', I mean just that: I am continually surprised that so many running fans actually manage to look so miserable while they are supposed to be enjoying themselves. Skimpy shorts in biting cold weather, a hang-dog expression and bright pink nose do not exactly add up to an inspiring sight. Personally, I feel that all forms of sport should be enjoyable and that includes running. I find it a good way to ensure basic stamina and endurance wherever I happen to be, even if it is miles away from the nearest sports arena. I try to run at least once a day. I endeavour to pick the most interesting routes and, if possible, run with a mate or mates who will help set the pace and inspire me to keep going! And, if it is cold, I wear a warm, comfortable tracksuit or tights under shorts – not just running shorts and T-shirt.

To get the maximum benefit from running, you should remember that the muscles you use actually go through a relatively small range of movements, and repeat the same basic actions. Therefore, to increase the benefits, you should aim to do different kinds of running – fast, slow, uphill, downhill – and have a break or breaks during the run for a set of exercises and a quick rest. That way, you will do the greatest amount of good in the shortest possible time, and give your body a total workout, not just an endurance test with the clock as your master. Of course, if you are a budding marathon runner, it will be necessary to keep a strict watch on your performance – monitoring your time, pulse rate and breathing, plus distance; but, for less ambitious runners, it is more important to ensure *regularity* than high performance.

Here are some tips:

CHOOSE YOUR CIRCUIT

Pick a park, attractive (and *safe*) road or track near your home, and make sure it is interesting enough to keep you coming back. I have several favourite routes: a park near my home in Surrey; a country run when I am in Crawley, Sussex; and a track at the New River Centre in Haringey, London. When I arrive anywhere – whether it is a sports meeting venue or not – I immediately look for a suitable running circuit. It could be a stretch of beach in the

Seychelles, or a leafy suburb. I actually prefer to run on grass or through woods and I am lucky enough to have had the chance to run through some of the loveliest scenery in the world. However, I still enjoy coming home to my local circuits – and you will find that, if you run on the same route regularly, you will be entertained by the changing seasons, the flowers, trees, architecture and people you meet *en route*. It will become a very personal part of your life – a place where you can switch off mentally while you tune up physically.

WEAR THE RIGHT GEAR

As I have already mentioned, the correct running shoes are essential, and the clothes you wear should be loose and comfortable (see chapter 2). Jeans are just not flexible enough for running and the elasticised kind can restrict movement and lead to muscular cramp. A warm tracksuit, or warm tights and shorts plus tracksuit top, for winter – cool shorts, and T-shirt, or a light cotton tracksuit in summer, are ideal. Socks should be a good quality synthetic or cotton mixture, to absorb perspiration and prevent sore feet. For women the right bra is essential, and if you are a 75 (34″) or more, wear a cotton bra with wide straps – not too tight – and back which is comfortably supportive. In winter, it may be a good idea to wear a cosy woolly hat. If you run on holiday beware of setting off wearing a bikini or trunks. That early morning jog from your hotel in the cool breeze could turn into a sizzling slog once the sun gets high. So, cover up with proper running clothes and wear a sun visor or peaked cap to protect your head and eyes. I always wear a T-shirt in hot countries 'cos I'm shy!

Dehydration could also be a problem, so make sure your route passes by a good watering spot or take a flask of water with you. For both sexes, some kind of protective or moisturising face and lip cream is a good idea; in winter, wind can rapidly dry your skin and in summer you really do need sun-screen protection. I have a real problem with sun-burn in hot countries and always wear a sun-screen when running in the sun. What do I think about wearing a walkman? Fine, if you are not in a traffic zone. Personally, I would rather listen to the banter between the boys and myself, or the birdsong and my own thoughts – though music is great on other occasions.

CHOOSE THE RIGHT TIME

No, you do not have to get up at dawn every day! You should choose a time which fits in most easily with your own schedule. For working people, it is most beneficial and easiest to run after work and before starting evening activities – the run helps you switch off and refreshes you for the next part of your day, whether it is coping with the family or meeting your mates at the pub. Families can usually work out a routine together: dad to look after the children while mum has a run at 6 p.m., mum to cope with breakfast while dad has his run in the morning. If you are very tied-up with young children, get a friend to share the load – you mind his or her children while he or she minds yours, and vice versa. Later, the children can join in.

Lunchtime running is also good – if you are in the kind of job where it is practical to change into your gear and steam off to the park at 1 p.m. You really do need to have good washing facilities, though – preferably a shower – which you can use when you come back from your run. Teachers, factory and office workers with a set lunch-hour would probably find it easier to get into a running routine than those in jobs where meal-times vary, or where lunchtime entertaining is part of the job. Friends of mine who run after work say that the exercise makes them *less* likely to overeat at supper time (the additional oxygen intake gives the brain a 'boost' which makes hunger pangs diminish), and that a run is far more relaxing than a couple of pints at the pub on the way home.

What I must emphasise is that it is necessary to run *regularly* to feel the benefits: at least twice, possibly three times a week or, better still, every day. A once-weekly run is better than nothing, but it could also be dangerous if you slacken off considerably in between, and then run hard without a sufficient warming-up period first.

DO YOU ALWAYS NEED A WARM-UP?

I warm up by starting my run very slowly – so slowly, in fact, that most people *walk* past me at this point! However, if your time is limited and you aim to do a fairly fast run, you should make sure your muscles are warm and limbs supple. Do not do such a frenzied warm-up that you are too exhausted to enjoy your run. A few simple movements like these are adequate:

1 Arm and leg stretches

Stand straight, shoulders relaxed. Now raise your left leg behind you, left arm up and backwards. Stretch up and back as far as you can, looking up. Hold briefly, lower, then repeat with the other arm and leg. Repeat total movement five times.

2 Lunges

Stand straight, feet together, hands on your hips. Now step forward with your right leg, left leg straight out behind and legs wide apart. Make sure your weight is evenly distributed between your two feet. Now, bend your right leg, moving the weight on to it. Keep your back straight and get as low as you can without leaning forward. Bend and straighten five times, then swap legs and repeat.

3 Running on the spot

Do a few running paces, on the spot, and establish your rhythm and breathing before you set off.

PACING YOURSELF

If you have not been running regularly before, start by alternating walking with running: about 100 walking paces, followed by 100 running. If you are using a street circuit, you can use lampposts to pace yourself – walk between two, then run between the next two, and so on. Stop, if you feel tired (I stop even if I do not feel tired). As you run, do not think about the circuit ahead, just enjoy the moment itself. Gradually increase the running paces until you can comfortably run about half a mile without stopping. The time it takes to achieve this will depend on your starting fitness level – under no circumstances try to overdo things, and if you feel like going back to the running – walking routine for a while, do so. You may find that you experience a 'second wind' sensation when things suddenly become much easier, and your body feels lighter and stronger. This is quite normal and a really good sensation – top long-distance athletes often experience a 'third' or even 'fourth' wind.

RUNNING STYLE

Use the *balls* of your feet and let your arms swing naturally in an easy style. Do not swivel your pelvis

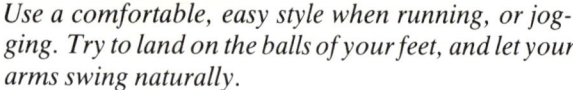

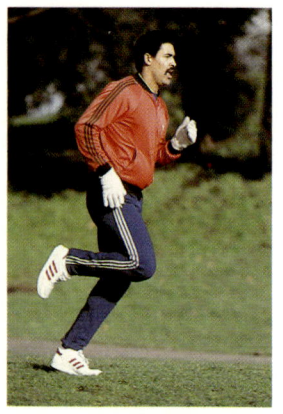
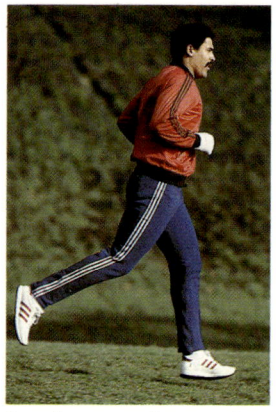
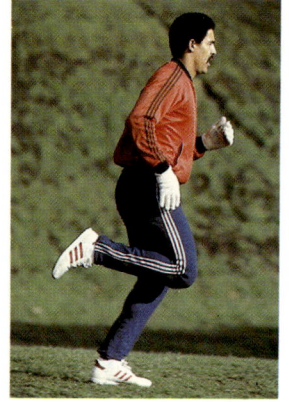
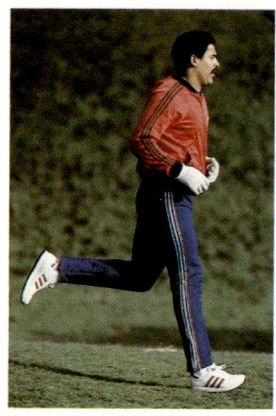

Use a comfortable, easy style when running, or jog-ging. Try to land on the balls of your feet, and let your arms swing naturally.

Pace yourself sensibly – do not try to go too far, or too fast. Do not swivel your hips, wobble your bottom, or turn your feet out.

or turn your feet out. Many women find that, when they start running anyway, they tend to run on their *toes* – this is because they have shortened Achilles tendons as a result of wearing high heels. Frankly, you *will* experience aches and pains after the first couple of runs, but a warm bath will soothe you and you will find that the creaks will soon disappear with regular running. Do not swing your arms too high – you will be making extra effort for nothing. Just be natural, comfortable, and you will soon develop your own style.

THE HALF-WAY STAGE

Aim to finish the first half of your run (the half-mile stage for beginners) at an interesting spot where you can do a simple exercise routine before setting off home. If you wish to run further than one mile and are fit enough to do so – then gradually increase your distance. One of the great pleasures of running is that improvement is a very rapid process indeed for

It is important to get rid of neck tension, so try some head circling first.

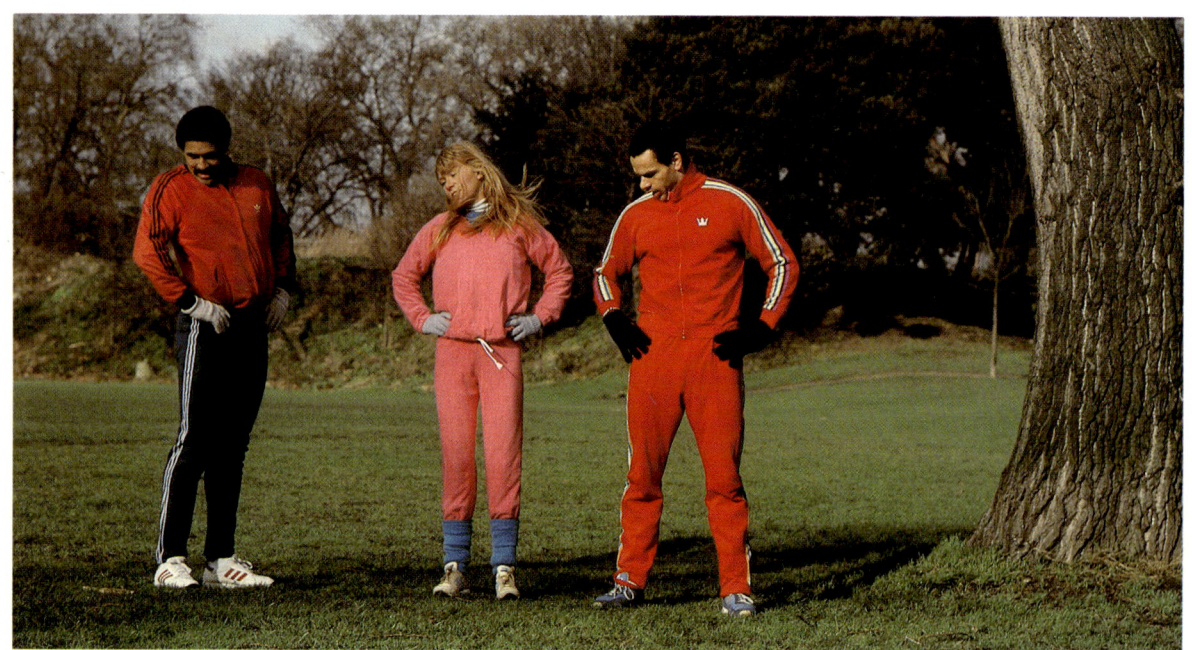

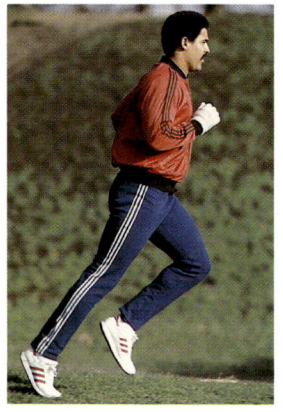 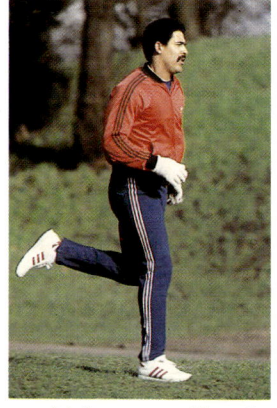

Do not let those arms swing too high – you will make extra work.

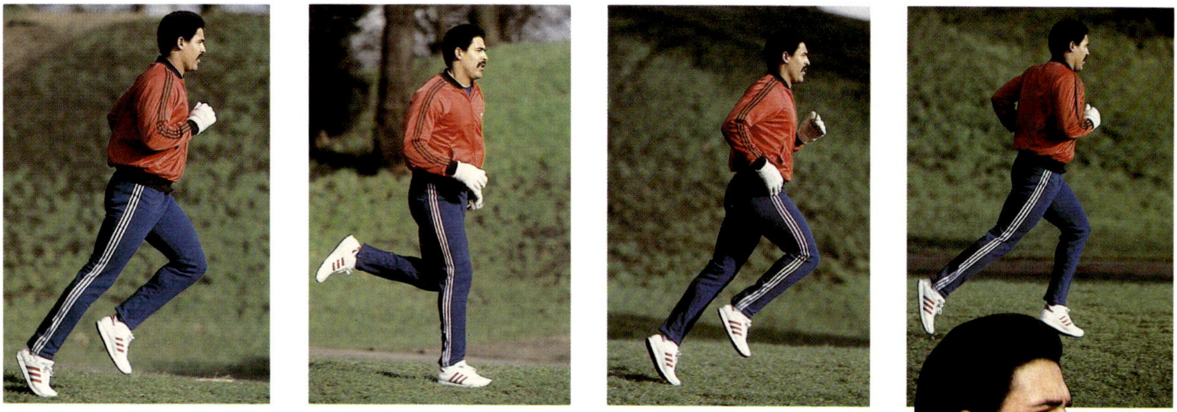

beginners (old, experienced athletes like me have to work very hard indeed over a long time just for a small improvement), so that you will soon feel able to cope with increased effort. Do not push things, though – an injury or muscle strain could interfere with your job and put you off running.

Here is a good exercise routine for runners, which is the one I generally use when I am doing my regular daily runs with my training colleagues:

1 *Head-circling*

Do this slowly: start with chin down, then turn your head clockwise, so that your chin touches your shoulder, then push your head back as far as possible, touch the other shoulder, then back to the front. Repeat five times each way to help release any shoulder 'knottiness' – do not *hunch* your shoulders.

2 *Side stretches*

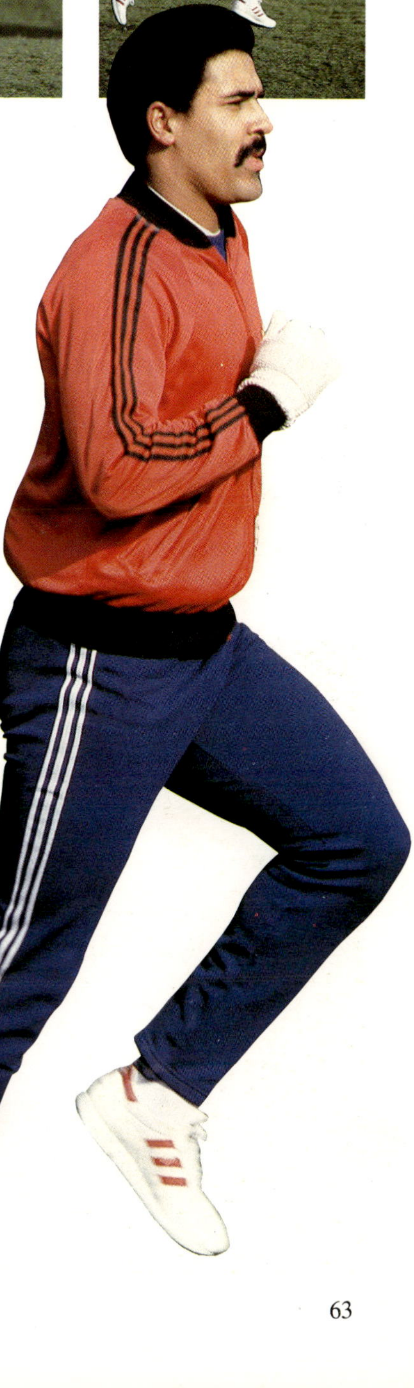

Stand with feet about 90 cm (3′) apart, arms by your sides, back straight. Curl your left arm, hand tucked

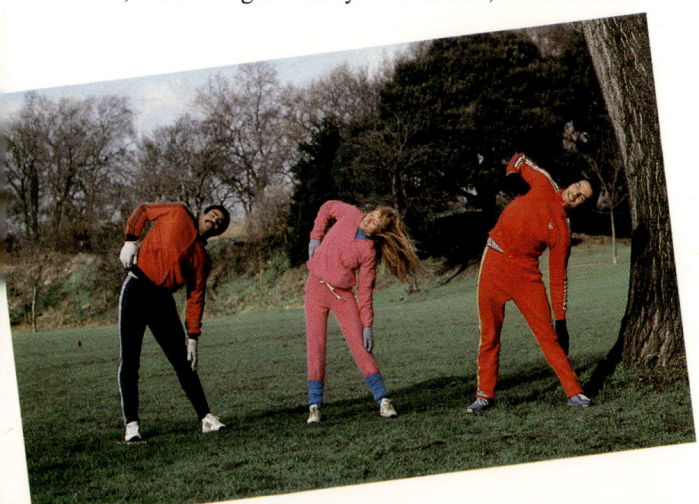

under, and lean over to the right, letting your right hand creep down your leg. You must keep your torso in a straight line – no spine twisting. Go down as far as you can, then straighten up – no 'bouncing', either. Now go down to the other side. Repeat the whole movement five times.

3 Arm swings

Stand straight, feet about 90 cm (3′) apart, hands crossed in front of you with palms facing your body. Now raise your arms and swing them backwards, palms upwards, drooping your head back slightly

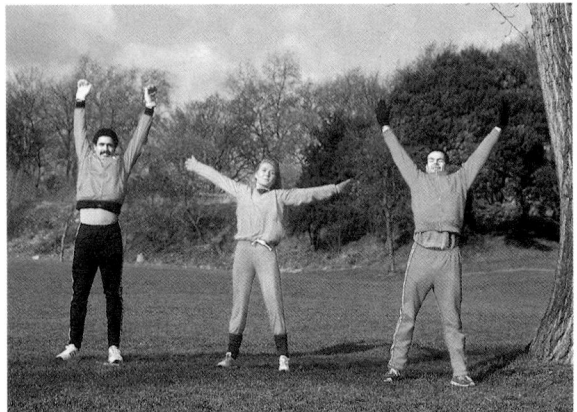

when hands are above it. Stretch up, but do not raise your heels. Lower hands to first position. Repeat five times, swinging arms up and down.

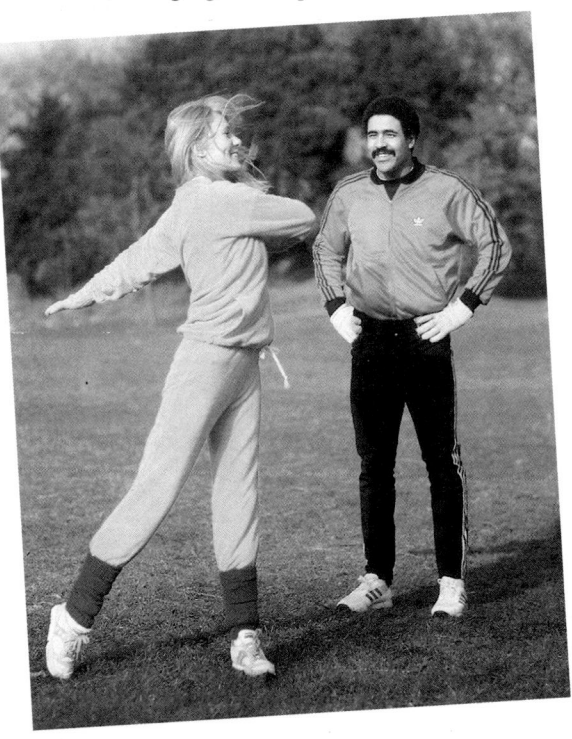

4 Torso twists

Stand straight, feet about 90 cm (3′) apart. Now raise right arm to chest-level and bend your elbow, so that your right hand is straight, palm down. Raise your left arm horizontally to your shoulder. Now swing round, from the waist, toward the right, keeping your arms level, and raising your left heel off the ground. Go as far as you can, then return to starting position. Repeat to the other side, then repeat the whole exercise ten times more in a continuous movement.

5 Hip circles

Stand with feet 30 cm (1′) apart, hands on your waist. Now circle your hips, forward, to the side,

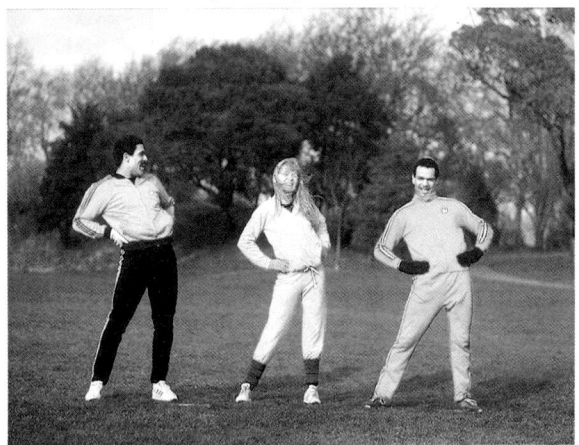

back; first to the left, then to the right, keeping your stomach and bottom tucked in. Repeat ten times each way.

6 Leg swings

Stand at arms' distance from a tree or wall, using both hands to steady yourself. Now swing your left

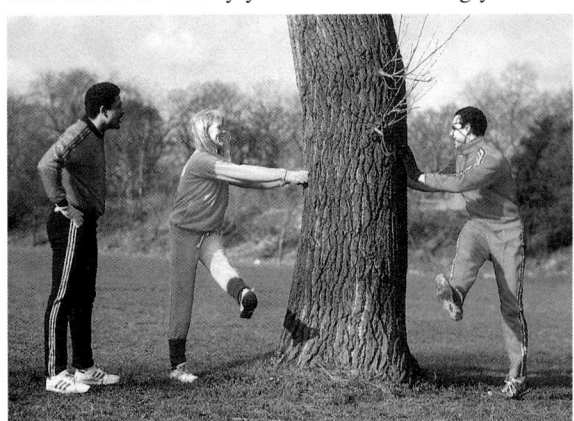

leg forwards, then backwards ten times, going as far as you can. Now swing it out to the side, then down and across to the other side, ten times. Repeat with right leg ten times.

7 *Calf stretching*

Turn to face the tree, about 1.2 m (4′) from the trunk. Now place both hands on the trunk, arms

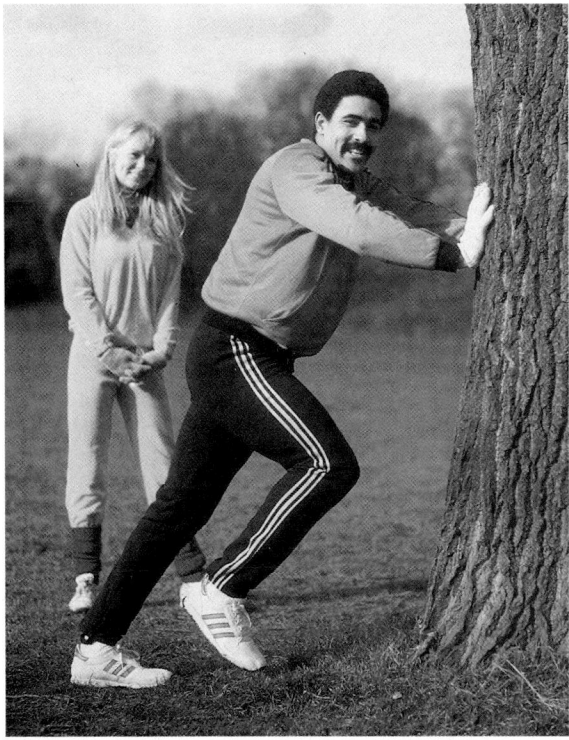

straight, and lean forward. Bend your left leg, raising your left foot off the ground, and lean forward a little more so your right leg is 'stretched', right heel on the ground. Repeat five times, swap legs and repeat.

8 *Hamstring stretch*

Now stand straight, cross one foot over the other,

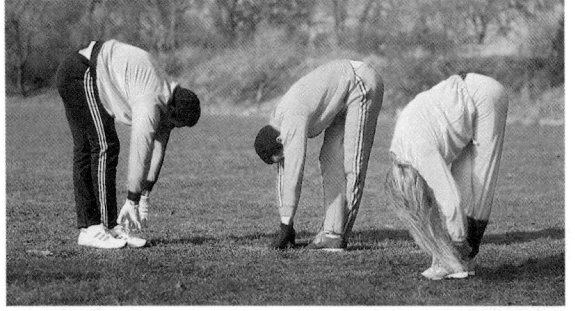

and try to touch your toes – your front leg may be bent, but keep your back leg straight. Do not jerk or strain – just go down very gently. Repeat twice, then cross legs the other way and repeat.

9 *Foot circles*

Now use the tree for balance while you raise first one foot then the other and circle your foot carefully, clockwise and anti-clockwise, about ten times each way.

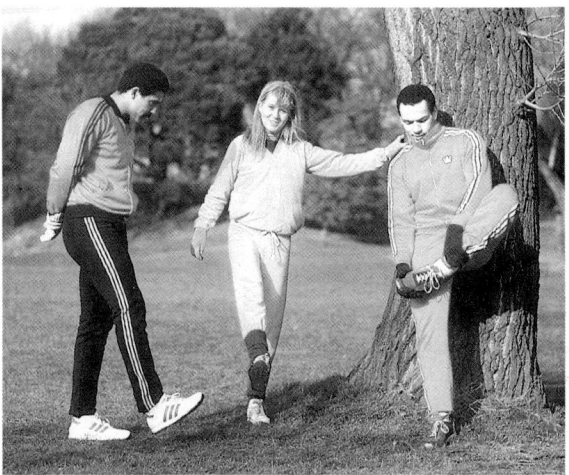

TRAINING FOR DISTANCE RUNNING

If you have ambitions to become a marathon runner, then you must approach your training with determination – but, whatever happens, never lose your sense of humour about things!

First, I would advise you to start a diary, with a daily entry detailing distance, and/or time, terrain, the way you felt. Do not start off by buying a stop-watch and trying to run a bit faster every day – you will simply become exhausted and may even injure yourself. Instead, alternate fairly tough and easy periods: for instance, if you go for a fairly fast six-mile run one day, drop down to a slower-paced three-mile run the next day. Aim to increase your *weekly* running mileage total very gradually to give your body and mind time to adapt to the new discipline you are demanding. It makes sense to plan your campaign *backwards* from the event, allowing a more gentle routine directly before the event itself. This is how I plan my own training schedule before a big sports meeting.

Be prepared to notice the changes taking place in your body as your efficiency increases: if you take your pulse rate and blood pressure before and after training, you will notice that they both return to normal more quickly as fitness improves. You will find you can run comfortably taking in less oxygen – breathlessness becomes less of a problem as you improve.

Because I am a great believer in having *fun* while I train, I would probably include the Swedish *Fartlek* method of marathon training if that was my event. This method (it means 'speed play'), developed by Gosta Holmer, who was chief coach of the Swedish 1948 Olympic team, consists of alternate fast and slow runs over different terrains with the accent on *fun*. For instance, a ten-mile training session could involve running through wooded country, over hills, sprinting through a shallow stream, then a slower-paced jog, followed by a fairly fast run. I believe that this kind of training really does help develop endurance, stamina, and distance – and it can always be alternated with more controlled distance running sessions round a track or on fairly even countryside. It prevents *boredom*, which is to be avoided at all costs!

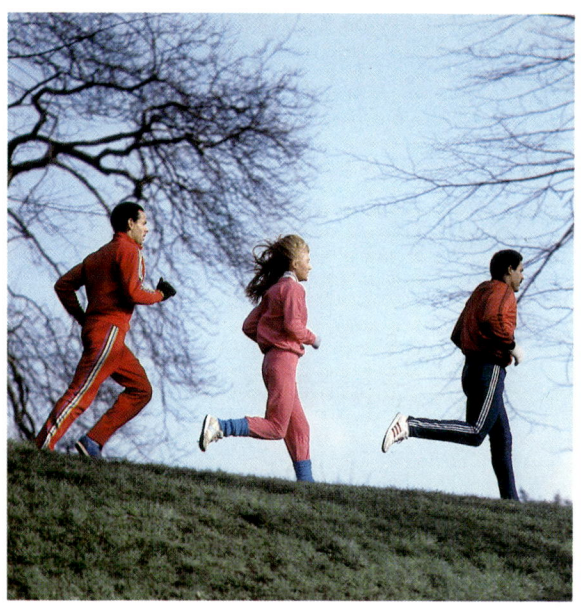

Running is such fun that you may find you travel further than you think! Goodbye. . .

DIARY OF A DISTANCE RUNNER

WEEK ONE

Monday 1 hour easy running over golf course.
Weather: windy. Felt tired at beginning.

Tuesday Jog 15 minutes
45 minutes easy *Fartlek* (strides and jogging to recovery).
Weather: showers. Felt relaxed.

Wednesday Jog 15 minutes.
10 or 12 × 400 metres. Rest of 200 metres between.
Weather: cool. Easy at first.

Thursday 1 hour easy running along seafront.
Weather: showers, strong wind. Tired.

Friday 30 minutes jogging, early morning.
Weather: cool. Nice n' easy.

Saturday 2 hours long road run, hilly course.
Weather: warm. Tired, but pleased.

Sunday 1½ hours running on golf course.
Weather: warm. Felt stiff at first.

WEEK TWO

Monday 15 minutes jogging.
10 × 100 metres up steep hill.
Weather: heavy rain. Quick hard session.

Tuesday 50 minute *Fartlek* on golf course and in woods. My favourite running.
Weather: cool. Felt relaxed.

Wednesday 10 minute jogging.
3 × 1 mile at a good pace with 5 minutes rest between. Ran in woods on firm paths.
Weather: windy. Last mile very hard.

Thursday 1 hour easy running at below marathon pace.
Weather: showers. Knee hurting.

Friday Rest.

Saturday 2¾ hours long running over mixed terrain, road, paths, woods and grass.
Weather: sunny. Knee OK. Felt strong.

Sunday 1½ hours easy *Fartlek* on golf course.
Weather: fine. Felt wonderful.

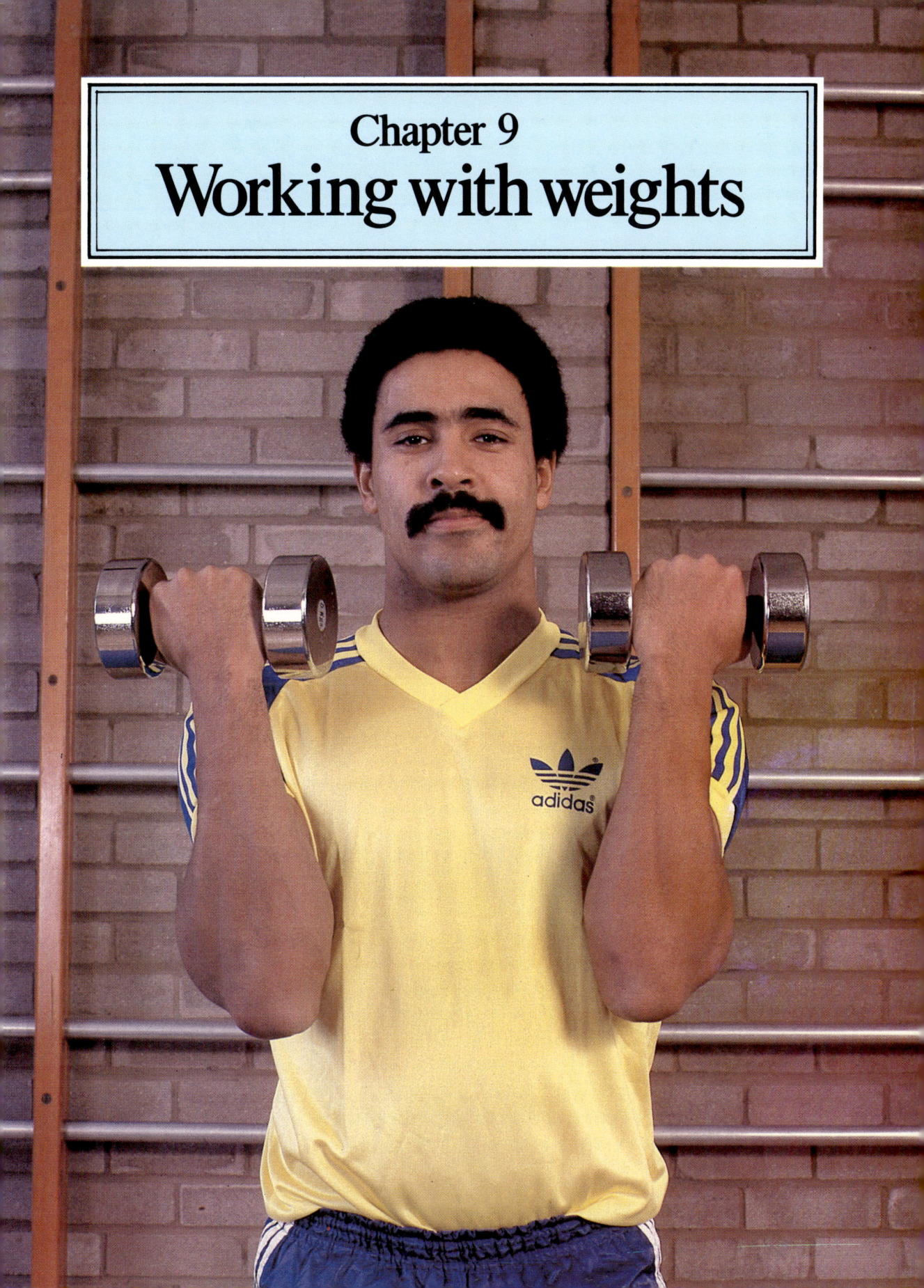

Chapter 9
Working with weights

TRAINING WITH WEIGHTS

Weights are useful for training for many sports, and can help improve your standard and give a welcome variation to your training programme. Actually, the 'throwers' in athletics (which include the hammer throwers, as well as my own three throwing events) do come quite close to Olympic weightlifters in strength requirements.

Sprint runners can use fairly low repetition, fairly high poundage general exercises; and high repetition, low-poundage work is good for long-distance runners. Swimmers can use dumb-bells to help build up arm strength, and foot weights for their legs (the East German Olympic swimming team spend almost a quarter of their training time working with weights). The same goes for ball game enthusiasts, even golfers – I know that many of the top class players work out with weights to keep in trim. If you are involved in a sport which demands sudden fast sprinting effort – such as cricket, lacrosse, basketball or netball – weight-training can help make certain that your leg and back muscles are up to producing the maximum effort when it is required. Finally, I recommend weight-training for those with hidden physical strength requirements, such as racing drivers, motor bike fans, horse-riding enthusiasts, and yachtsmen.

WHAT WILL WEIGHTS DO FOR YOU?

But what about those who want to keep in trim and improve their figure and general appearance – will weight-training just develop huge muscles and make the ordinary man or woman turn into a Mr or Miss Universe? That is a common misconception about the whole principle of working with weights. Very simply, weights help to increase the force of contraction of a muscle, building up strength so that the muscle can do the job of helping efficient, strong body movement. As the weight load is increased, the muscles work harder – but it is only with a really massive work-load that the muscles become so enlarged that they look huge. An ordinary person doing weight-training using fairly light weights would never, ever build up this kind of superman look! As so many muscles are involved in even the simplest of movements, very simple weight exercises can have a good effect on many muscles, which means that weight-training is an economical as well as an effective way of working out.

Does it help you slim? You really need to combine weight-training (as any other exercise) with a sensible diet to lose weight, but you may certainly find that your body measurements change even if you do not alter your diet. By encouraging weak muscles to strengthen up, you are discouraging fat deposits from forming – this can be particularly noticeable around the abdominal, thigh, and upper arm areas after a concentrated weight-training programme. My friend and weight-training adviser, former decathlete Snowy Brooks, now teaches exercising with weights to men and women at a London exercise studio, and he has had very encouraging results on figure improvement for both sexes.

Women who want to improve their bustline have noticed that pectoral strengthening exercises help to give their breasts a 'lift', which makes them look higher and firmer. Men who have flabby stomachs notice very rapid firming and strengthening – particularly if they do weight-training at lunchtime instead of drinking in the pub! If you are too thin and want to look chunkier, weights really will not have any dramatic effect, unless you work hard at building up muscles by increasing the load progressively. But the training will give you more confidence and certainly help improve your general shape.

USING WEIGHT MACHINES

Weight machines are equally good for men and women – and very useful if you have only a short time available for your training. If you are interested in using weight machines, you must make sure that you have an instructor to show you how. If you work out in a gym, you will probably get the opportunity to use machines which work on specific muscle groups. One good system is the Nautilus. At present, Nautilus is available at only a few health clubs in Britain (other, less sophisticated, systems are used in most gyms), but is widely used in America. I use Nautilus to help increase my shoulder flexibility for javelin. Each machine (and they all look like instruments of torture!) forces a certain muscle or set of muscles to use its full range of motion against resistance. It also exercises the appropriate joints. Make sure you start off with the machine geared to a fairly light resistance (you can easily increase the load later), and do a warm-up before going on to the machines; never use them with 'cold' muscles.

WORKING WITH WEIGHTS

WHAT KIND OF WEIGHTS SHOULD YOU USE?

In the gym, you will find bar-bells, weight machines, dumb-bells, and the new Nautilus equipment, which I am demonstrating in the photograph on the next page. These are all variations on the basic theme of weight-training. Get the right instruction before you plunge into a programme, and make sure that your very first routines are supervised properly, so that you know you are doing the exercises correctly and using the proper weights for each movement. If you are doing the training as part of the build-up to an event or competition in some other sport, it is important to keep a diary of progress and get expert advice on the most useful exercises and best weights to use. Even if you are simply weight-training for fun and fitness, it is a good idea to monitor your progress on a record card and most good instructors will suggest this. The number of times you work out weekly depends on your time and what you intend to achieve with the programme, but try to use weights as a 'breather' between intensive training bouts, with three or four workouts weekly for serious sports people, two for the less committed.

WEIGHT TRAINING FOR THE DISABLED AND INJURED

Weights can help strengthen the upper part of your body, even if you are confined to a wheelchair. Paraplegics include the bench press in their competitions, and the blind and partially blind already have their own weightlifting competitions. If you have been injured in some way which does not affect your general level of fitness (a broken leg, for instance),

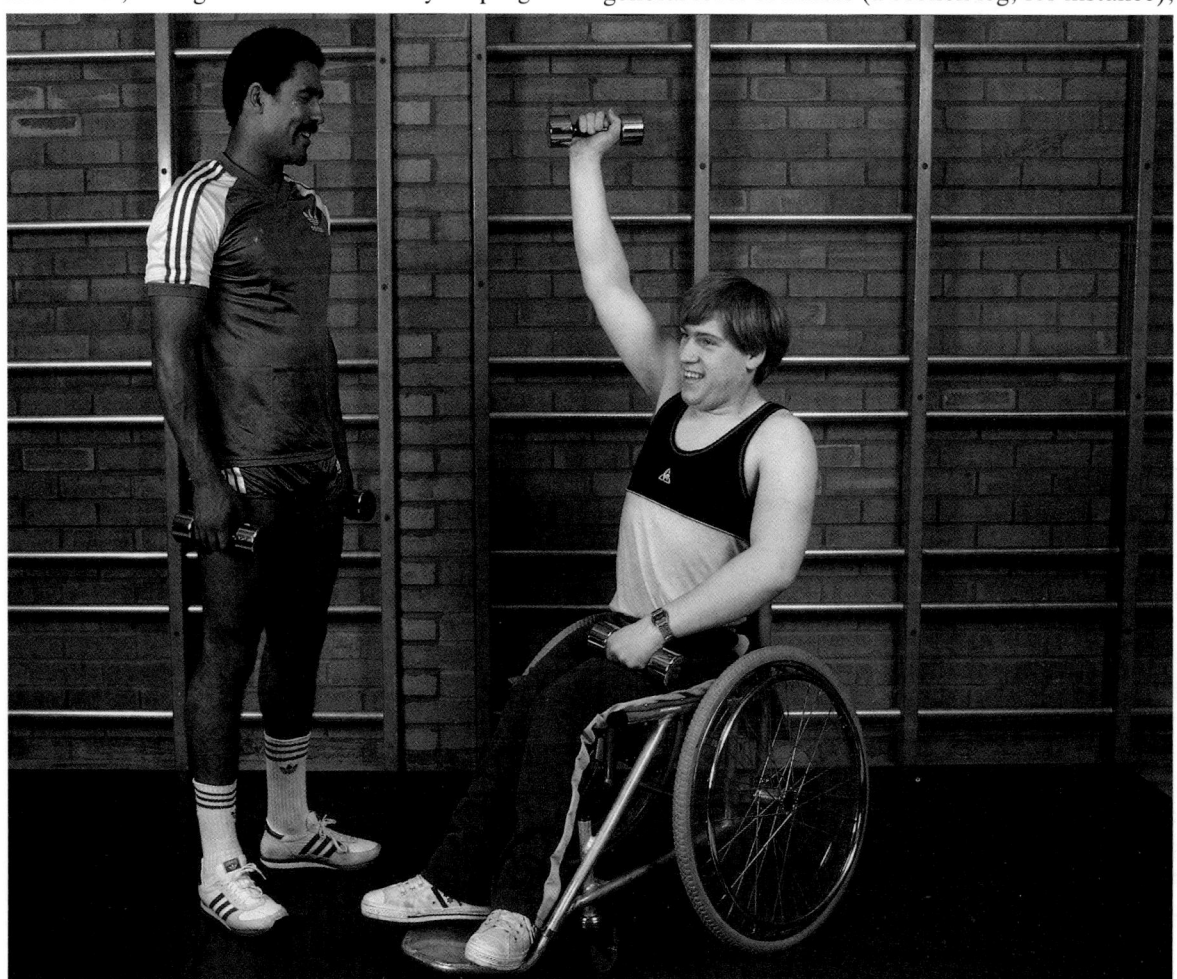

Disabled athlete Jamie Gilham, 16, works out with weights every day

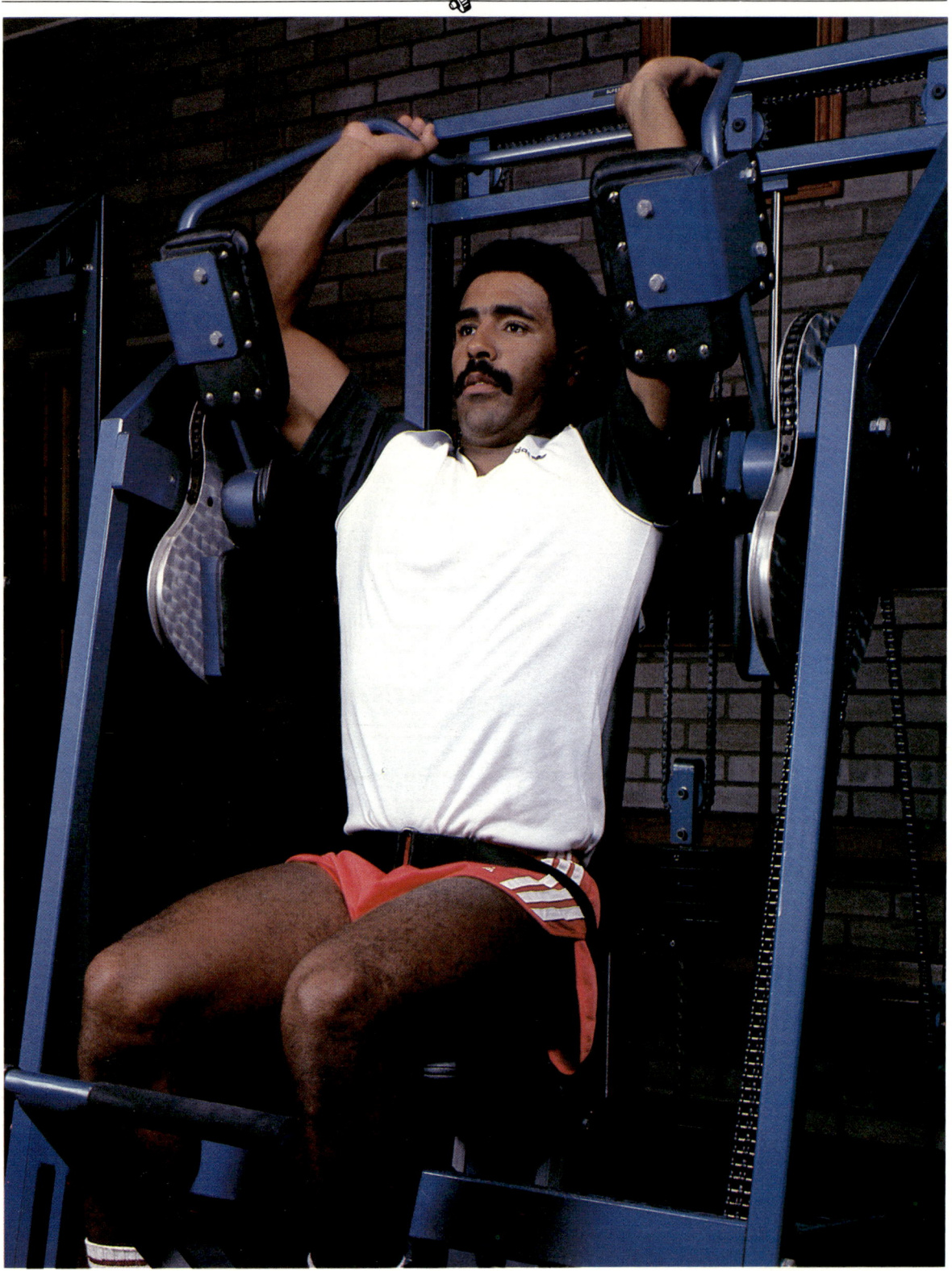

This machine is called a 'Pull Over', in the Nautilus system, useful for increasing shoulder mobility for javelin

you can use weights to ensure that the rest of your body retains strength and tone – but you will need a modified schedule which you should check out with your instructor or club coach. When your body is recovering from illness, be very cautious with weights; get advice from your doctor before resuming training, and use a lighter load than usual until you regain optimum fitness.

I know many athletes who have used weights successfully after illness to regain full sporting fitness more quickly than would have been possible without them, but they begin training only when they feel able to cope with simple exercises again. Barry Sheene, the brave motor cycle champ who recently underwent massive leg surgery to rebuild his shattered limbs, used weights to keep the upper part of his body in trim while recuperating, and then gradually included leg exercises as his legs became stronger. With the result that he was back in action far sooner than anyone imagined possible.

WEIGHT TRAINING AT HOME

Most weights – like bar-bells – are relatively expensive and cumbersome and must in most instances be used in the gym. However, dumb-bells are really ideal for your home training session, as they are reasonably priced to buy and easier to store. But, if you buy them, do beware of any exercise literature on the box in which they are packed – in many cases, this is not scientifically devised (often, it is very badly translated from German or a Scandinavian language with pictures which are not detailed enough for you to follow easily). Check out the exercises with an instructor before you embark on your home programme. You can also improvise with weights if you like, using tins of baked beans, treacle (make sure the top is secure) or even large-size beer cans (full!) in place of dumb-bells. Choose a 3 kg (6½ lb) weight first, and progress to higher weights as your strength improves. Some dumb-bells have the screw-on type of weights which can be adjusted. Personally, I prefer the all-in-one heavy metal type, which are smooth and comfortable to hold.

Here is a programme of exercises to try at home using 3 kg (6½ lb) or 5 kg (11 lb) weights, or one of the improvised weights. Please note that correct breathing is very important during weight-training. If you try to inhale and lift, your bodily function is resisting the lift. The process of exhaling, however, gives power to your lift. So remember, exhale as you lift, inhale as you lower the weights.

1 Alternate front dumb-bell raises

Stand straight, feet about 25 cm (10″) apart, with a dumb-bell in each hand. Your arms should be straight down with your palms facing your thighs. Lift your right arm over your head. Lower it slowly, at the same time raising your left arm. Make the

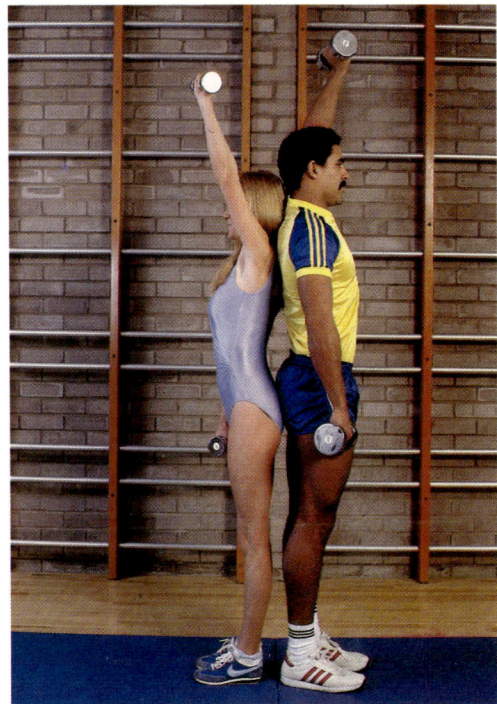

movement steady, moving the arms simultaneously, with the dumb-bells passing at shoulder height. If you have a friend who can do this one with you, stand back to back for additional back support. Repeat ten times with each arm. Do two sets increasing to three. This strengthens, tones and smoothes the shoulders.

2 Lateral raises

Stand straight, feet about 60 cm (2′) apart, a dumb-bell in each hand, with your hands by your sides at hip level. Lift your arms straight up to shoulder level, without bending your elbows, then let them back down again slowly. Repeat ten times, increasing to twenty-five. Do two sets, increasing to three. This works the shoulder muscles called the outer deltoids and helps eliminate excess flab around the upper arms and chest area.

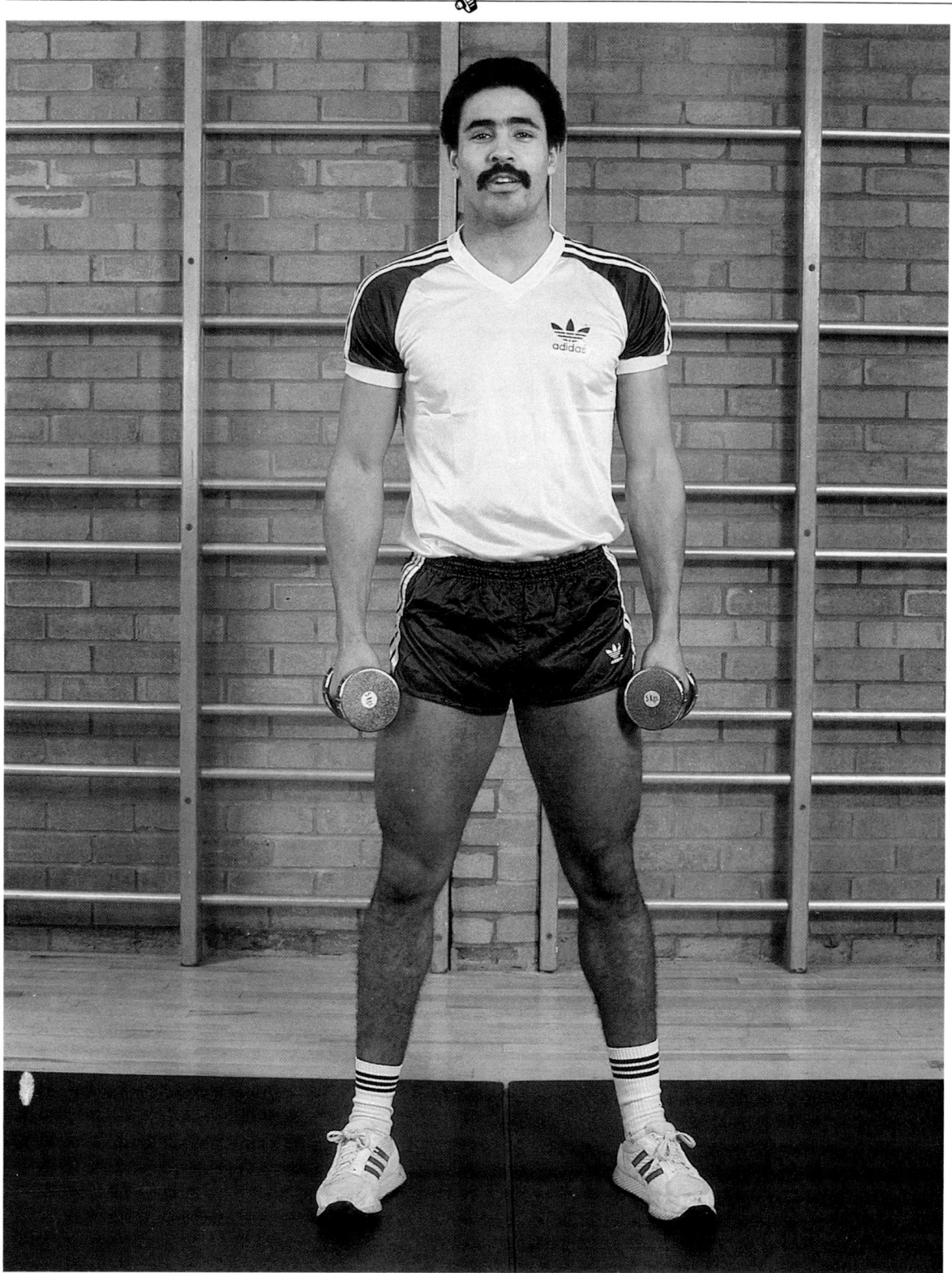

Lateral raises help eliminate flab around the upper arms and chest area

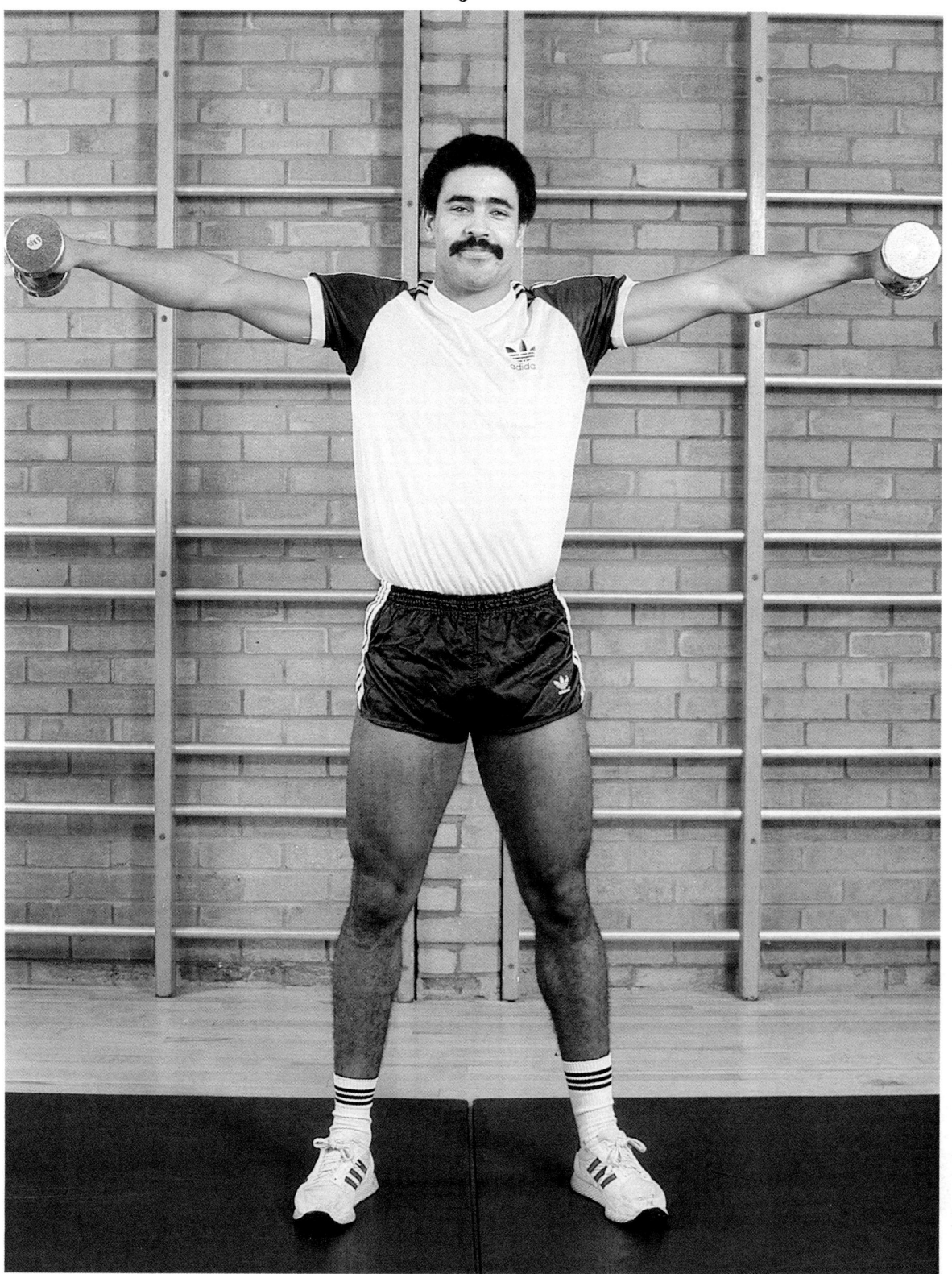

3 *Overhead press*

Stand with feet apart, hands at shoulder height with a weight in each hand, palms facing inwards. Now raise your hands right up above your head, pause briefly, then lower them slowly. Repeat ten times, increasing to fifteen. Do two sets increasing to three. This is good for arms, shoulders, breathing, chest.

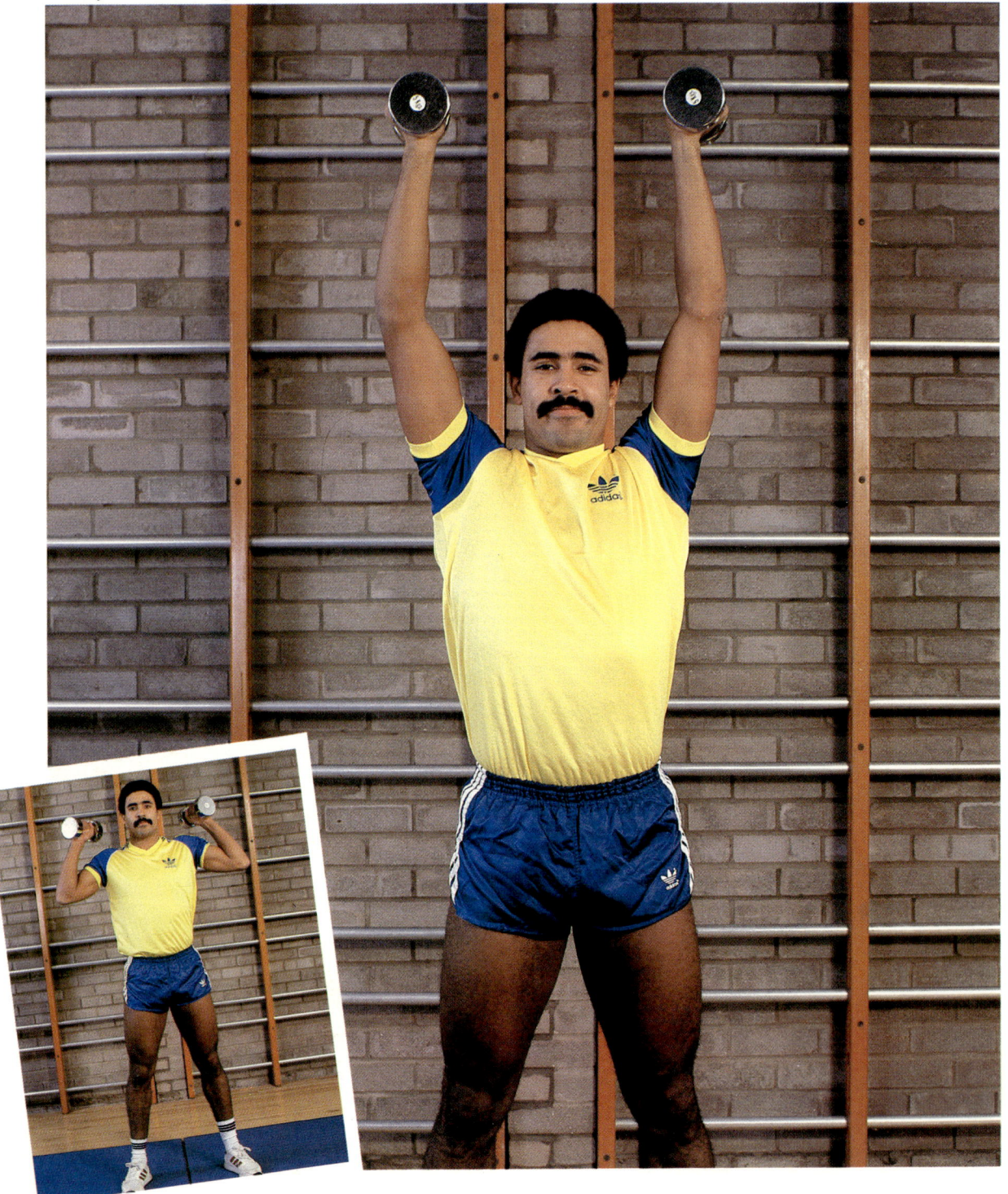

4 *Dumb-bell curls*

Stand straight, feet about 30 cm (1′) apart, with a dumb-bell in each hand, palms facing forward. Press your upper arms firmly against your sides. Now lift the weights, moving just your forearms until the weights come up to shoulder level. Very slowly, let the weights go back down to starting level. Repeat ten times. Do two sets, increasing to three. This tones and strengthens the bicep muscles in the upper arms, helping to eliminate flab and build up strength. Good for tennis, badminton, squash.

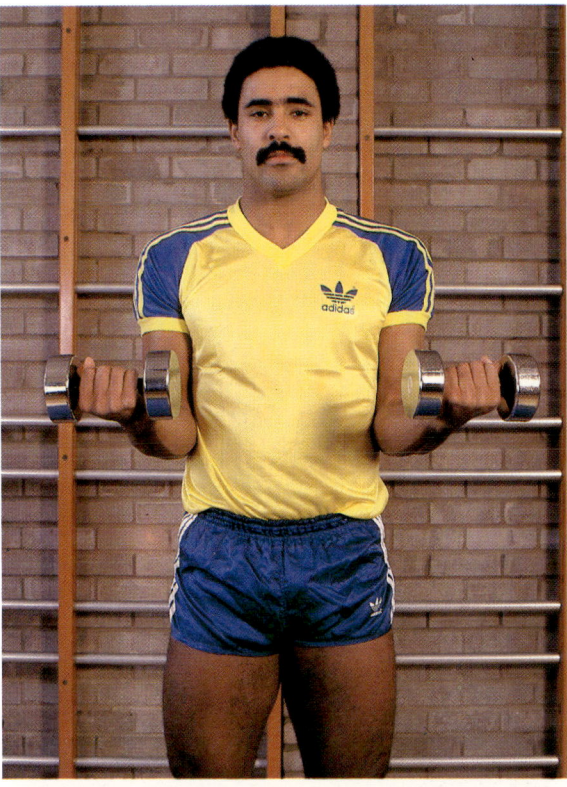

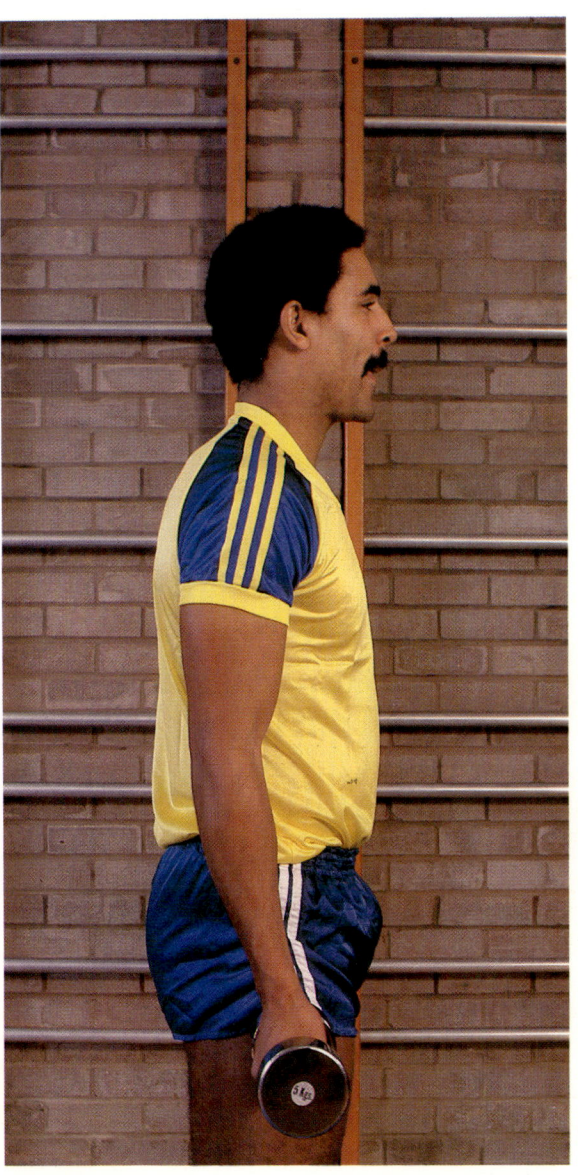

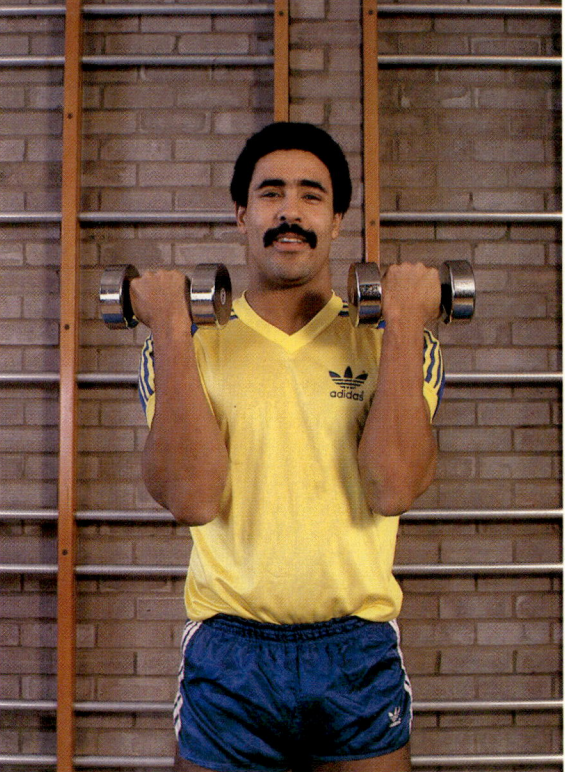

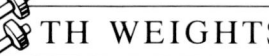

5 *Step-ups*

With a dumb-bell in each hand, step up and then down on a low bench or step (the front doorstep is ideal). Keep up the rhythm, with alternate steps, making sure your head is up, your back straight, for twenty steps, increasing to forty. Do two sets, increasing to three. This strengthens all the leg muscles, particularly the calves and the thighs. It is also good for general stamina.

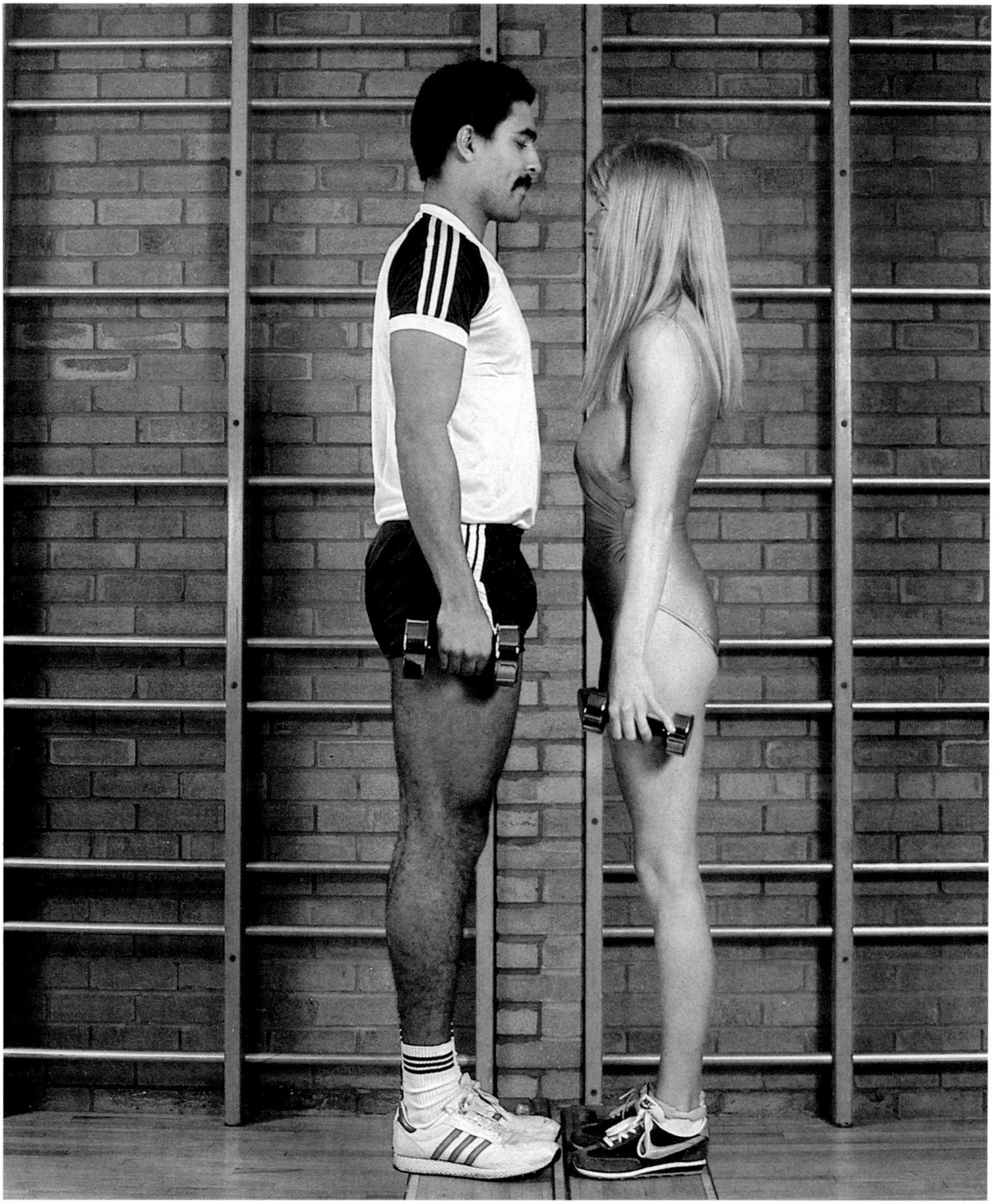

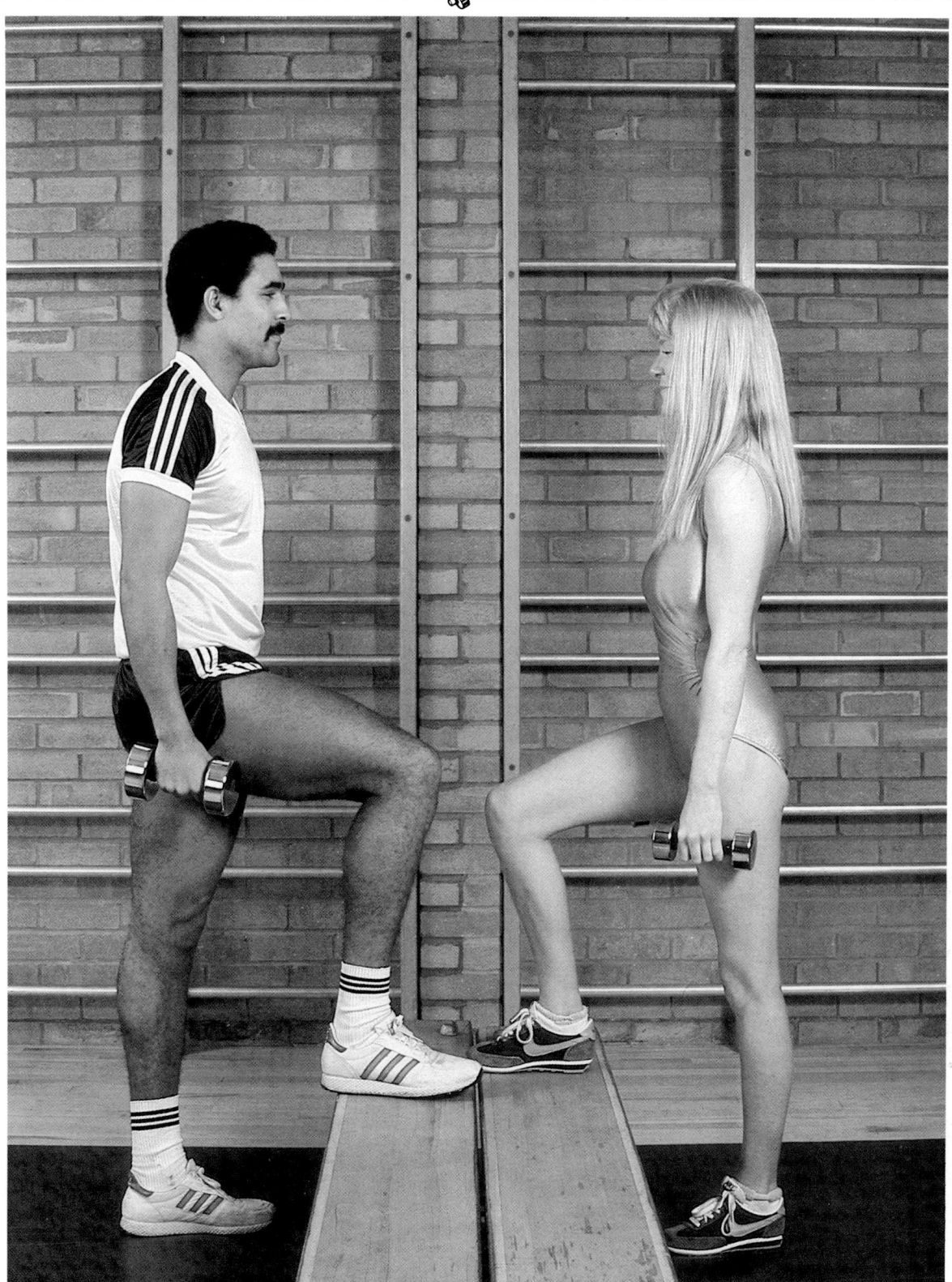

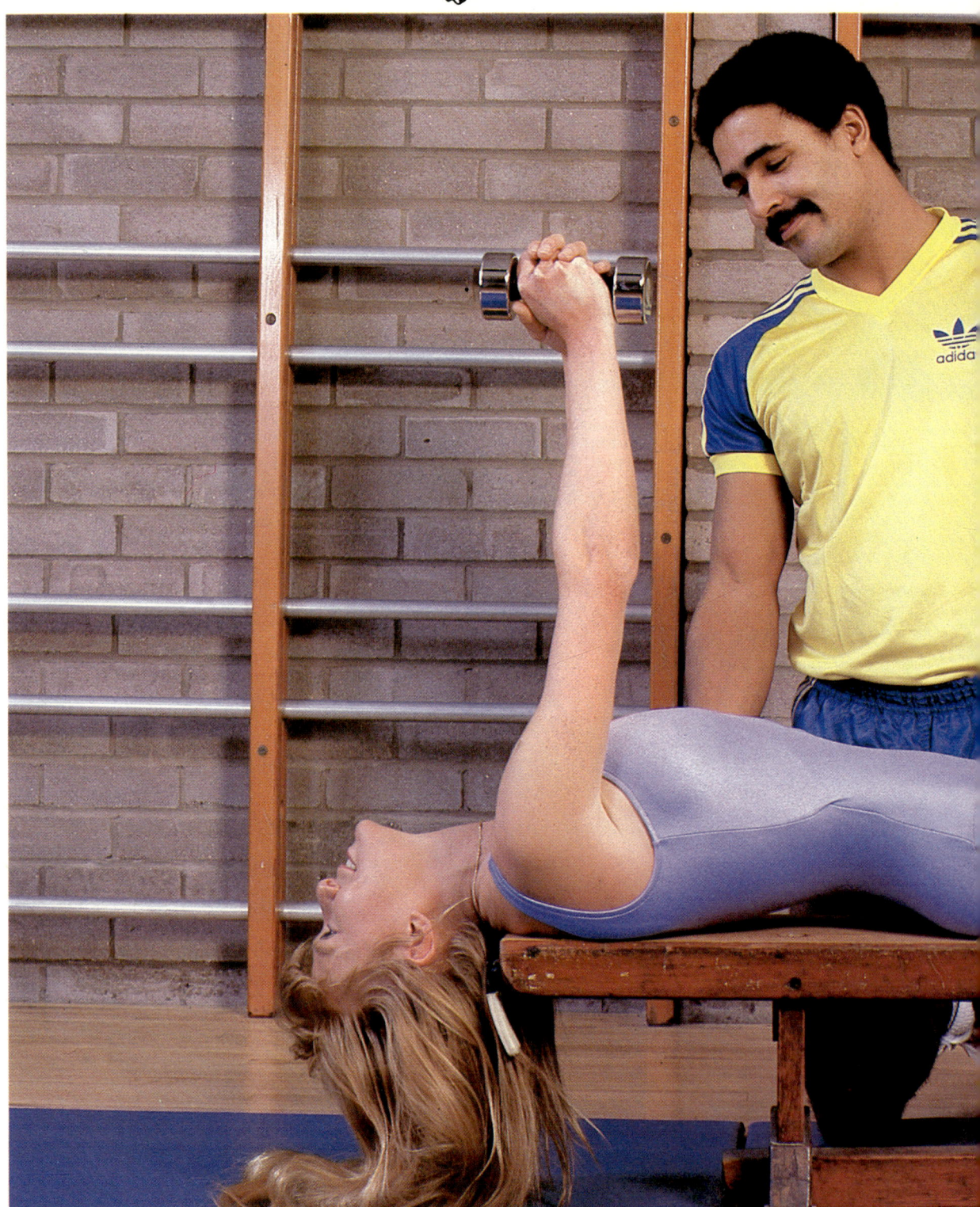

This exercise – pullover with dumb-bell – helps develop the pectoral muscles which support the breasts. Instructions on the next page.

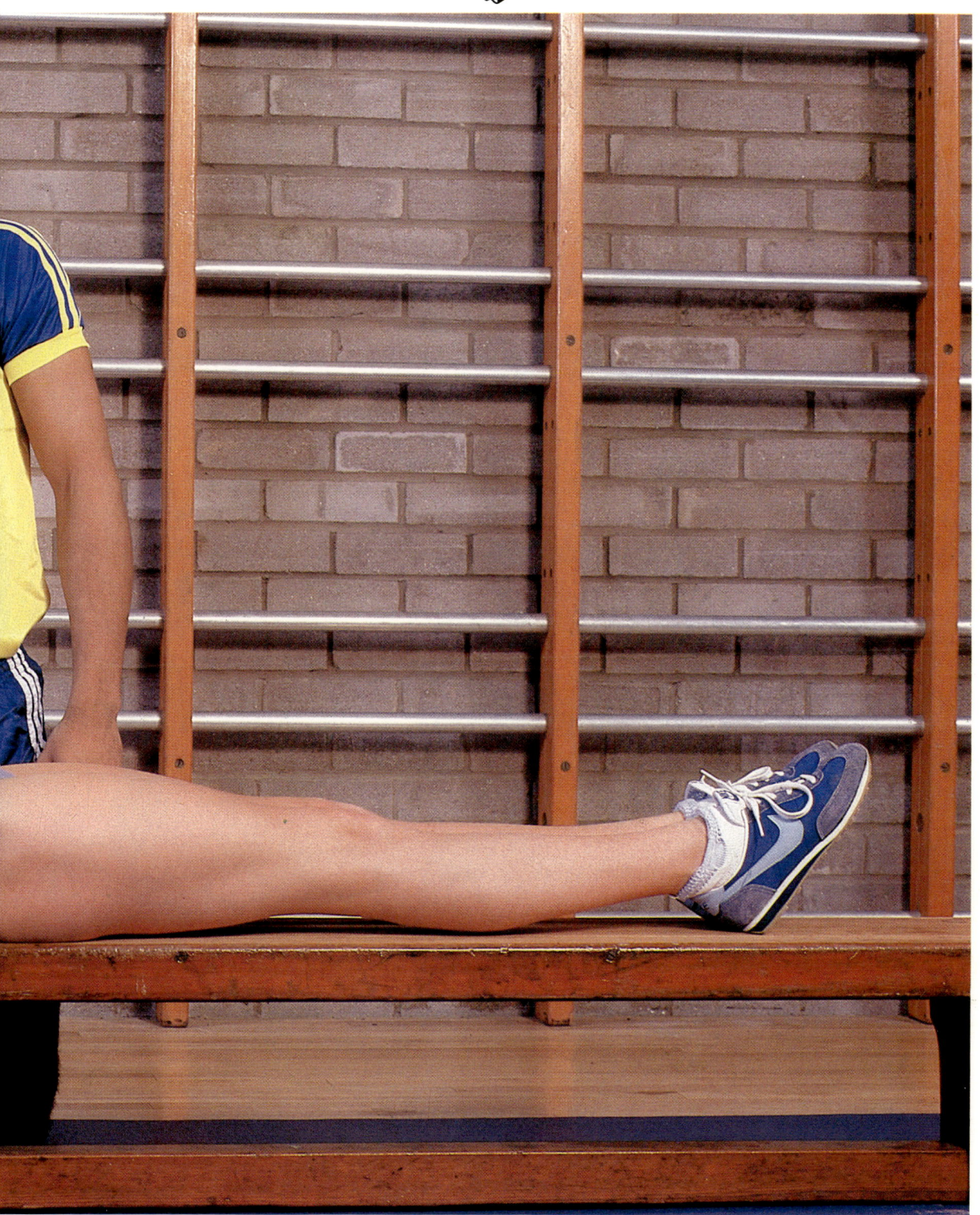

6 *Pullover with dumb-bell*

Lie flat on a bench or bed, with your head hanging over the end of the bench, the back of your neck adequately supported. Holding one dumb-bell in both hands, raise your arms straight above your chest. Now lower the dumb-bell down behind your head, keeping your arms straight and allowing them to go as low as possible using their own weight as leverage. Hold, then raise the weight above your chest once more. Repeat ten times, increasing to twenty-five or thirty. Do two sets, increasing to three. This is an excellent exercise for expanding the ribcage and improving your chest or bustline. It helps strengthen the pectoral muscles which support the chest.

7 *Dumb-bell bench press*

Lie on the bench or narrow bed, with knees bent, elbows bent, a dumb-bell in each hand. Push dumb-bells up, arms straight above chest, then bend the elbows and repeat ten times, increasing to twenty-five or thirty. Do two sets increasing to three. This is another excellent exercise for chest and arms.

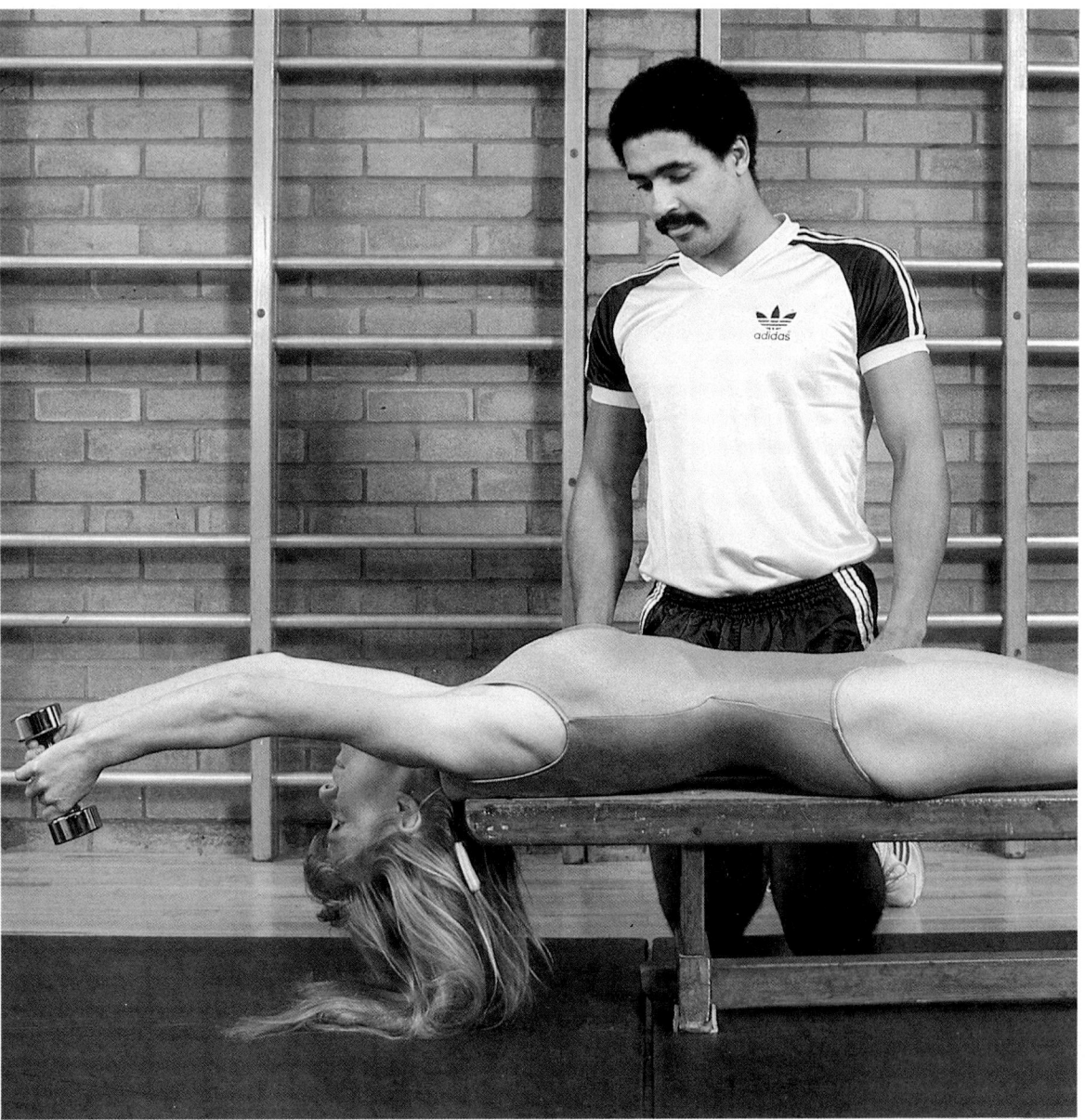

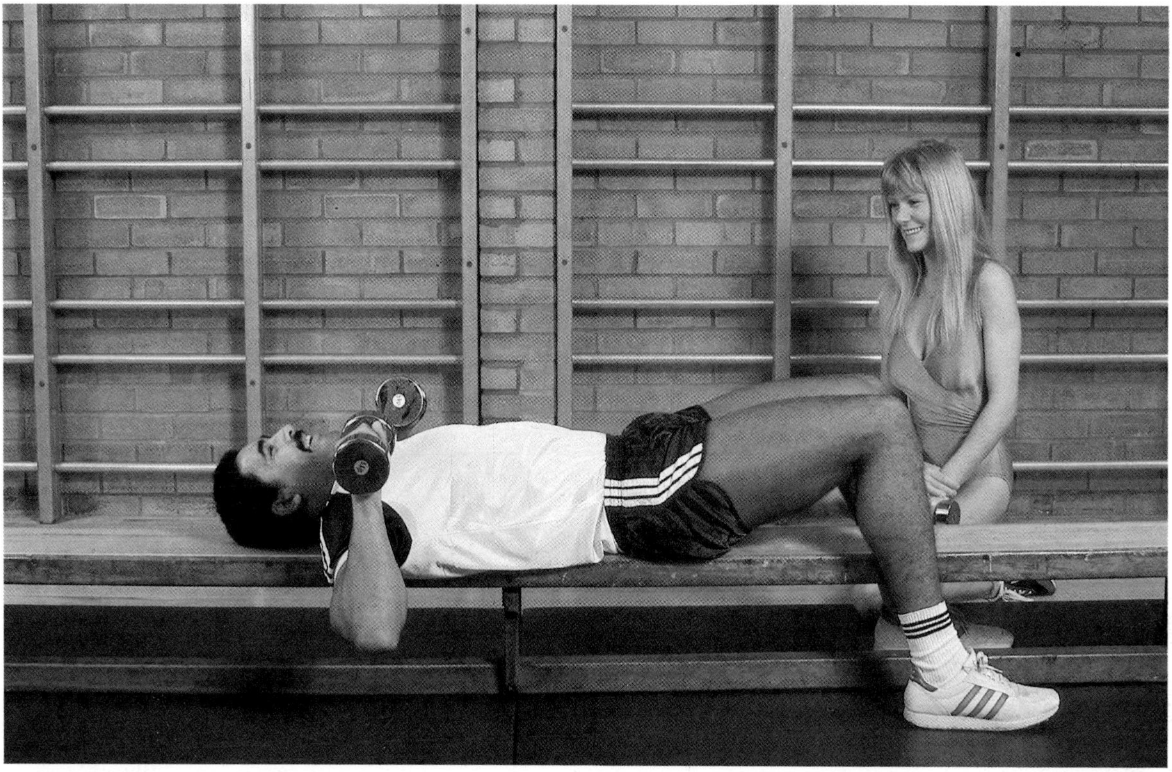

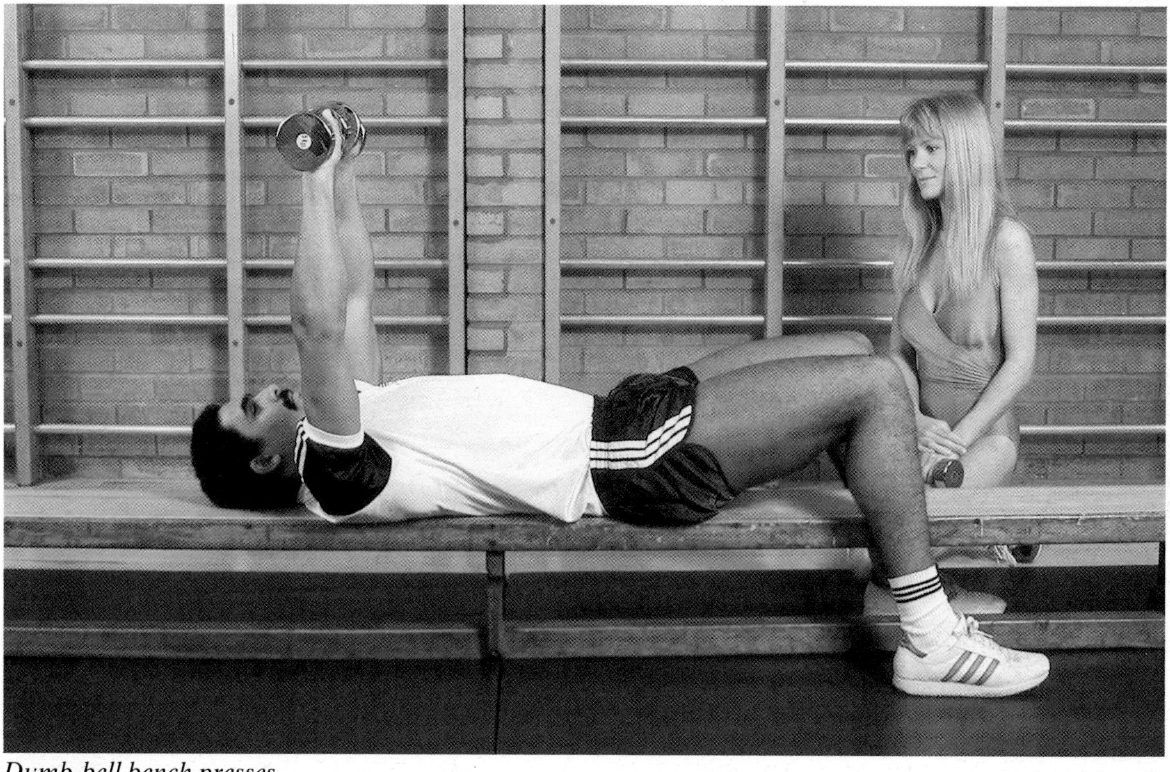

Dumb-bell bench presses

8 Squats

If possible, do this one in front of a mirror, so that you can check your posture. Stand with your heels on a book. Hold a dumb-bell in each hand. Now keep your upper body straight, and bend your knees, lowering yourself into a squatting position, until your thighs are parallel with the floor. Come up slowly. Repeat eight times. Do two sets increasing to three. Breathing – inhale on the way down, exhale coming up. This is a good buttock-firmer and thigh strengthener. If you gradually increase the load, you can build up very strong leg muscles for ski-ing, cycling or tennis with this exercise.

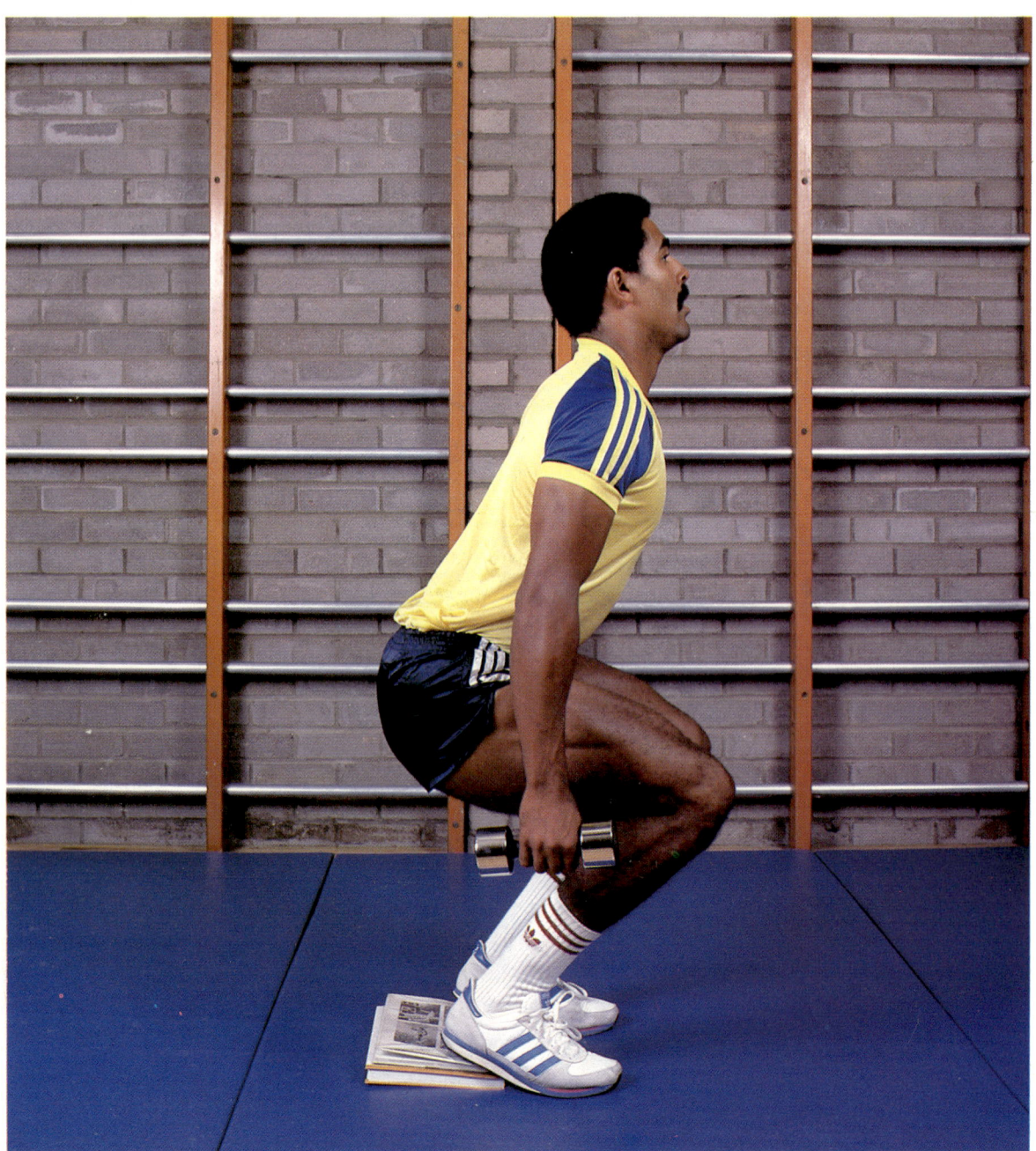

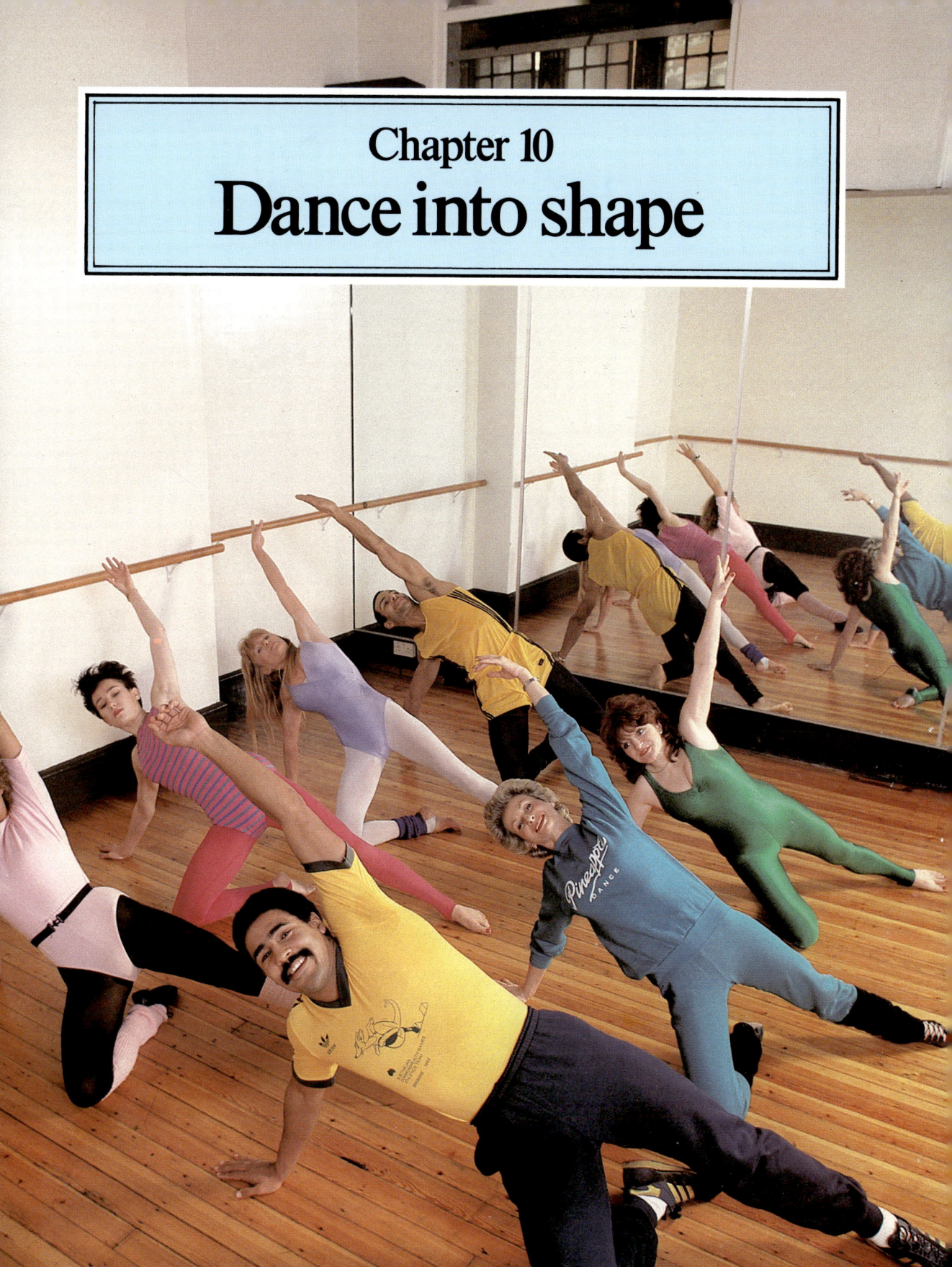

Chapter 10
Dance into shape

I have a secret ambition to join the Kids from Fame in one of their amazing dance routines – they look such fun and the dancers obviously have a wonderful time doing all those fabulous steps and almost acrobatic movements. But, I have to admit, that although I am a good mover, I am not yet up to that standard! Though I am sure they would be very patient if I joined in one of their rehearsals. There is a delightful natural friendliness about dancers and in dance studios that I am certain has contributed towards the popular explosion of dance-exercise. You only have to pop into a dance studio to be sure of good coffee, friendly faces, and a total lack of distinction between the professionals and the amateurs like me.

Recently, I spent a day at the Pineapple Dance Centre in London where teacher Sylvia Caplin is a living example of how ballet, exercise, music and healthy diet can do wonders for your figure and looks. Sylvia's ballet training, as well as her work with osteopaths, physiotherapists and doctors, have helped her evolve a method of exercising which is fun, easy, and really good for you – even if you have never been to an exercise class before. And that is the *real* test – for, sadly, there are some teachers who push beginners on too far (beware of being told to go for the 'burn', i.e., agony!), and who have little knowledge of basic anatomy. Do check out any teacher you go to before you attend the class just to make sure that she knows exactly what she is talking about. If she has a reputation for pushing students to the limit, opt out!

But do not let me put you off – for dance-exercise classes really are one answer for women and men in sedentary jobs or who spend time at home with children. Some sports centres now run dance classes in conjunction with crèche facilities which can be a real boon for mums and dads. Look on your dance-exercise class as a social event, too, when you can meet your friends (or the stars, or both!) and have some fun. There is a comforting anonymity about wearing a leotard or practice trousers and tops which makes everyone at the class feel at home – whether they are budding Nureyevs or mere decathletes with ambition!

MEN AND DANCE-EXERCISE

The vast numbers of books and records produced for women on the subject of dancing would indicate that men do not really go in for it. Nonsense. I believe that there will very shortly be a male dancing revolution with loads of ordinary guys leaping into the dance studios. At Pineapple, the installation of a gym has lured men in, and they are already joining in the classes. Well, fellas, I can heartily recommend dance classes as a great place to meet very nice ladies indeed!

WHAT DANCE-EXERCISE CAN DO FOR YOU

Immediate benefits of a regular dance-exercise session include less *stress*: you simply have to switch off everyday worries when you dance in order to concentrate on what you are doing. The increased oxygen boost also helps speed up metabolism, makes you feel brighter and more optimistic. You will probably find that you lose weight – the calorie-burning processes after a twenty-minute dance session are believed to remain active for two to three hours after the end of the session. The oxygen itself gives a 'high', so that you do not crave sweet foods after dancing. If you can remember to drink water or mineral water instead of sugar-loaded soft drinks after your class, you will avoid putting on compensatory calories and still quench that raging thirst.

Dancing has a marked effect on your body shape and bearing:

Posture and confidence

Because you really do have to throw yourself into a dance routine with abandon, you lose inhibitions very fast. Your posture is improved because your arms and shoulders get a good, relaxing workout, and your confidence increases. You find that everyday movements like sitting, standing, walking, become more graceful and controlled.

Breath control

Everyone huffs and puffs at first, but gradually you will find that your breathing is more economical and less gasping. This is very useful indeed for soccer and squash players, who need to expend their energy in a controlled way and breathe with maximum efficiency. I am sure that most Saturday League players would benefit from mid-week dancing.

Leg strength

Thighs, particularly, become stronger when you dance regularly, and you will find that other leg-strength sports like running and tennis will seem less tiring. Hamstrings and adductor muscles get a good, steady workout: hamstrings (at the rear of the thighs) by leg-stretching; adductors (on the insides of the thighs) by pointing the toe forwards and moving steadily on the spot. But make sure you do undertake all movements very gently indeed – do not strain yourself. Beware of doing the splits and straining your adductors which are also useful for making love, riding and swimming.

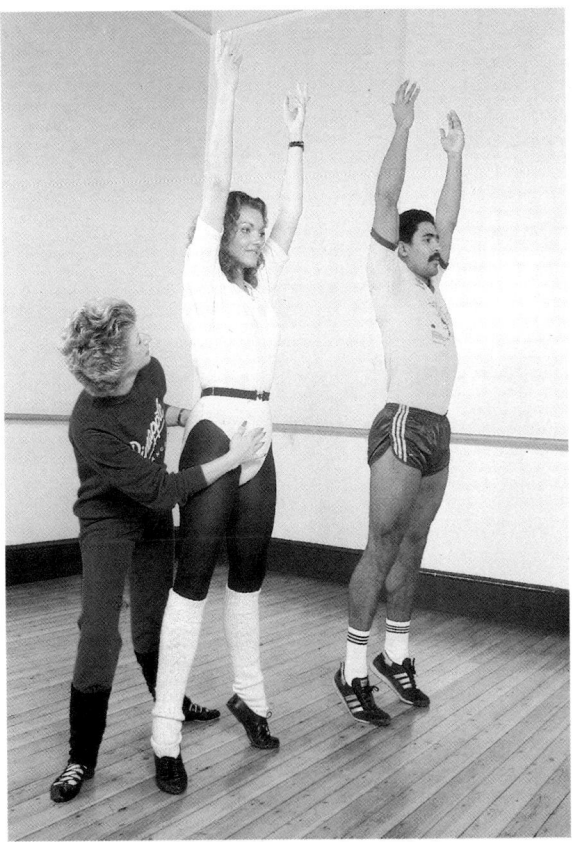

First check your posture

Stomach control

A good dance teacher will make sure that you stand well while you exercise (see Sylvia's posture exercise), and one of the benefits of this is an *involuntary* tightening of stomach muscles. By involuntary, I mean that you do it without thinking about it, and for most people who have spent their lives consciously trying to hold their stomachs in without much success, this is very cheering indeed. What is more, you find that, despite yourself, you are *still* holding in those stomach muscles several hours after the session.

HOW TO GET DANCING

Before you join a class, it is a good idea to practise some dance movements at home – not that you feel a fool in class if you do the wrong thing (after all, I managed), but you will get your money's worth if you are at least a bit used to moving to music. Keep up the action for as long as feels comfortable and fun, no longer. Although aerobic dance teachers stress the importance of maintaining a prolonged session to increase calorie burning processes and oxygen demand, I think it is dangerous to do a thirty to forty-five minute session straight away. Gradually, you can build up stamina, and technique, until a thirty minute programme becomes easy.

Age? Dancing is ideal for the very young, young, and not-so-young, but if you are worried about your weight, have a history of leg problems or respiratory disease, or have not exercised for many years, you really should have a check-up first.

Try these six simple exercises to some reggae or slow boogie, working up to a faster beat as you progress:

1 *Knees bend*

Stand with your feet together, arms out horizontally to the sides. Bend your knees to a count of four, bringing your hands down to touch them at the same time. Now straighten your knees, stretch up with your hands to a count of four, looking upwards to crossed hands over your head. Repeat this total movement five times.

2 *Side step*

Stand with your feet together, arms by your sides. Now step to the right, draw your left foot to the right foot, bringing your right arm forward, around and down to the right side, bending your knees slightly. Step to the left, draw your right foot to the left foot, bringing your left arm forward, around and down to the left, again bending your knees slightly. Repeat this movement six times.

3 *Body stretch*

Stand, legs apart, and look up at the ceiling with your back perfectly straight. Now reach up with your right arm, leaning into your right knee. Repeat with your left arm, left knee. Really *stretch* that body, looking up to the ceiling. Repeat twelve times each side.

4 *Walk it*

Now do eight walking steps to the left, bringing your knees up, and clapping your hands with each step. Repeat, with eight steps to the right.

5 *Bounce*

Stand straight, feet together, arms relaxed by your sides. Swing arms up to shoulder level, bend knees. Straighten legs, swing arms back to sides, with a bouncy movement. Repeat twelve times.

6 Repeat the whole sequence once – more as you improve.

7 Now go down into a crouching position, head tucked down, arms hugging knees loosely. Breathe evenly, stretch up, then lower arms gently.

YOUR MUSICAL WORKOUT

Concentrate on style, elegance and good posture throughout the workout, and do not strain. If you cannot quite manage some of the more difficult movements, simply go as far as you can – you will find that your suppleness improves with practice.

1 Before you start the routine, check your posture with this easy movement, which Sylvia Caplin recommends you use several times a day to bring your body into line instantly. Stand straight, feet slightly apart. Now raise your arms above your head, and go up on your toes. Pull in your stomach muscles, contract your buttocks and raise your pubic bone so that your pelvis is tilted forwards and upwards. Now raise your breastbone to elongate your ribcage, giving maximum room for breathing. This position should be held for a count of four, before you relax and start the exercises. If you do it in front of a mirror, you will see how much slimmer you look just by holding your body properly.

2 Lie on your back on the floor, knees bent, feet well apart, hands palms down on the floor beside you. Now breathe out through your mouth, exhaling and pushing the air out, while pulling your stomach in and pushing the small of your back into the floor. Inhale, letting your stomach expand. Repeat five times. Now relax for a few moments, knees down, feet together.

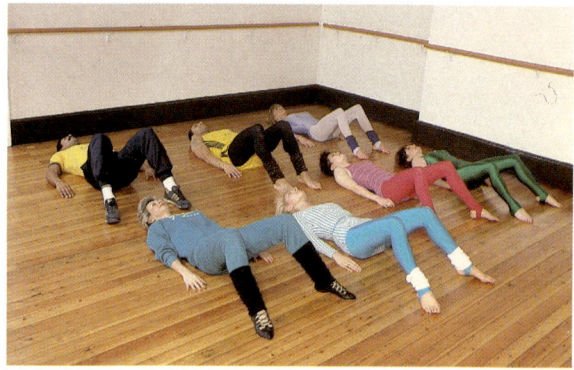

2 Breathe out through your mouth, pull your stomach in

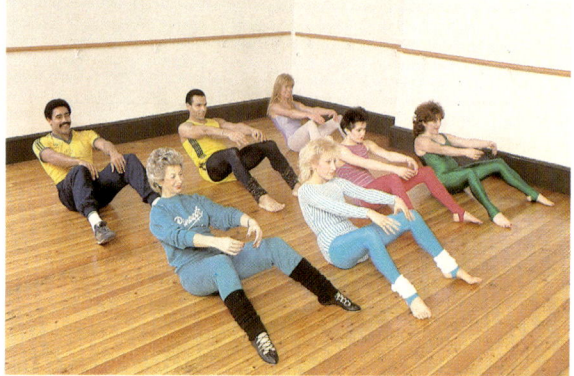

3 Let your stomach muscles do the work

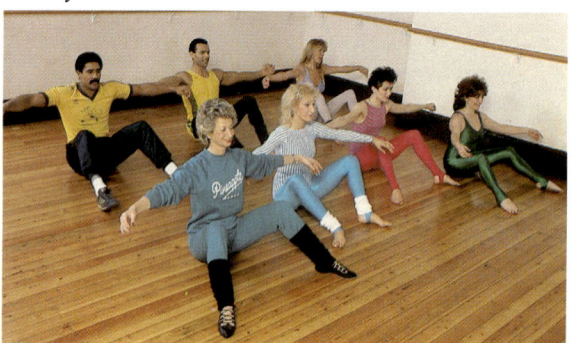

4 Move forwards on your bottom

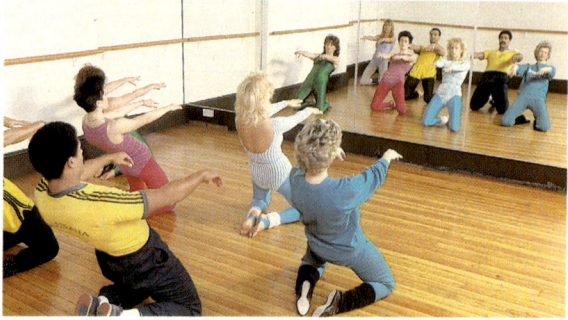

5 Lean back in a straight line

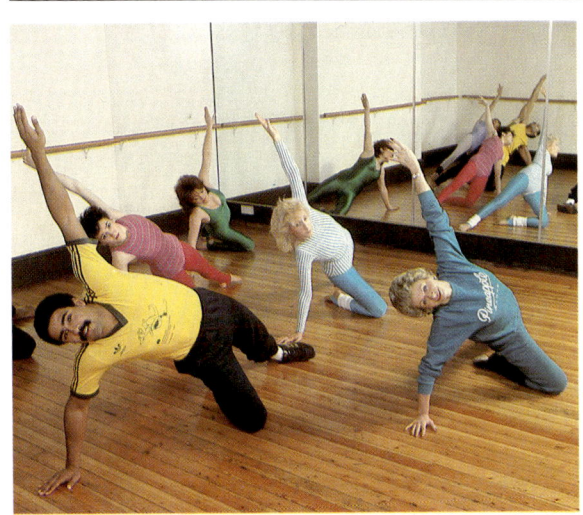

6 *Lean over and stretch*

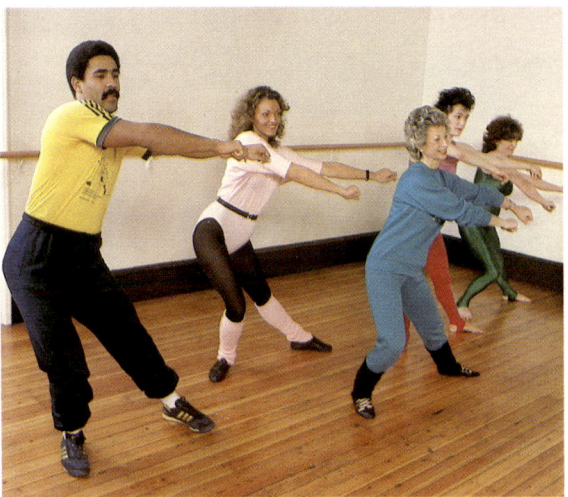

7 *Swing those hips to the right*

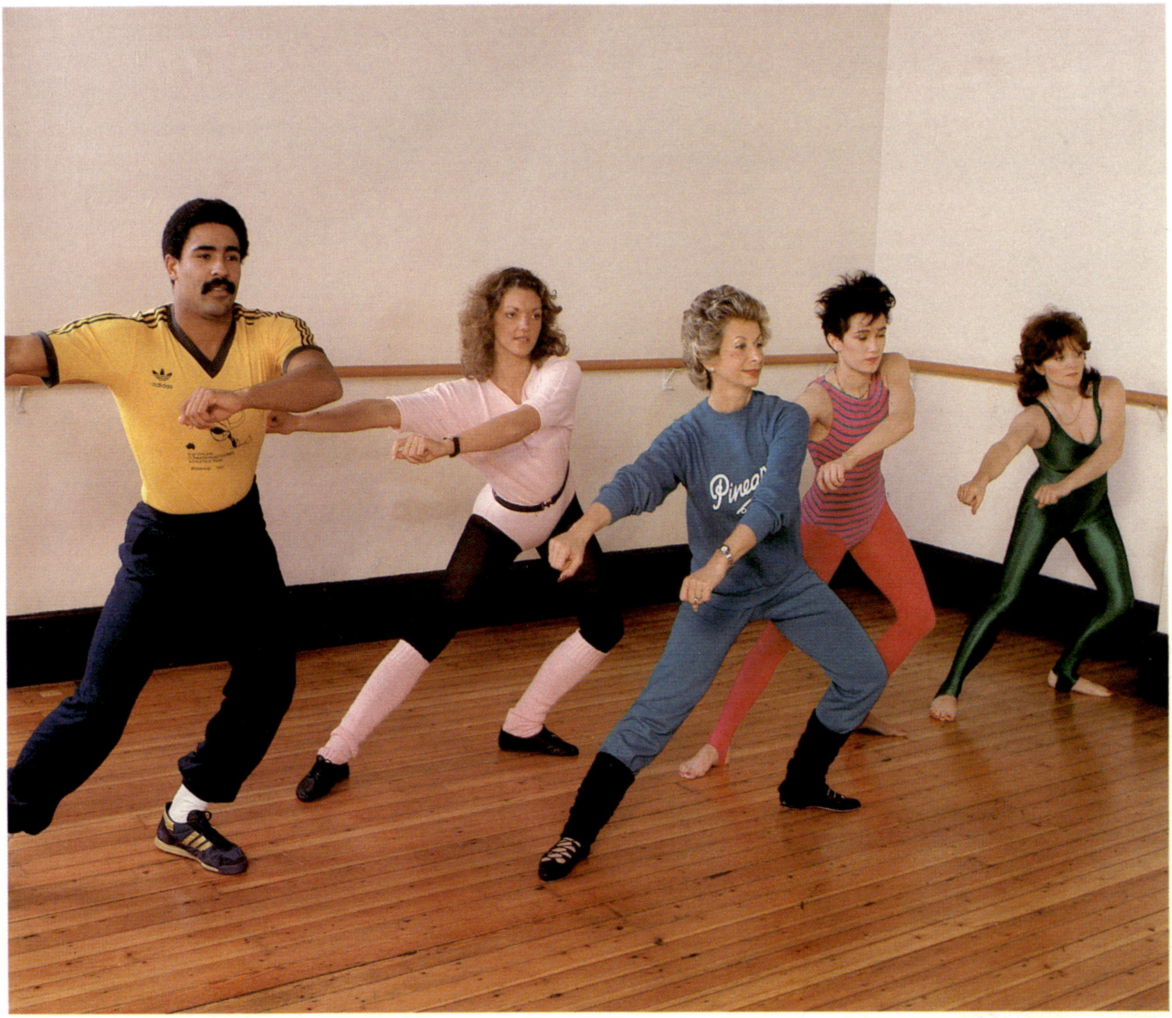

8 *. . . now to the left*

3 Knees up again, to the first position. Raise your arms, so that your hands are just above your thighs. Now pull in your stomach muscles and push forwards with your hands, raising your body off the floor (do not strain your back – your stomach should do the work). Push and push those arms through your knees, relax down again, push and push once more, aiming to get right up to the sitting position (you will not be able to at first). Repeat five to ten times.

4 Now sit up (use your hands to help raise your body, if you cannot make it without), still keeping those knees well apart. Arms out to the sides, palms down. Keep your back straight, pull in your stomach and rock from side to side on your bottom. Now shuffle forwards on your bottom, keeping that back straight, for a count of five.

5 Kneel up, knees well apart, feet together, hands straight out in front of you, palms down. Now let the top of your body lean back in a straight line, give a little bounce, then return to starting position. Repeat five to ten times.

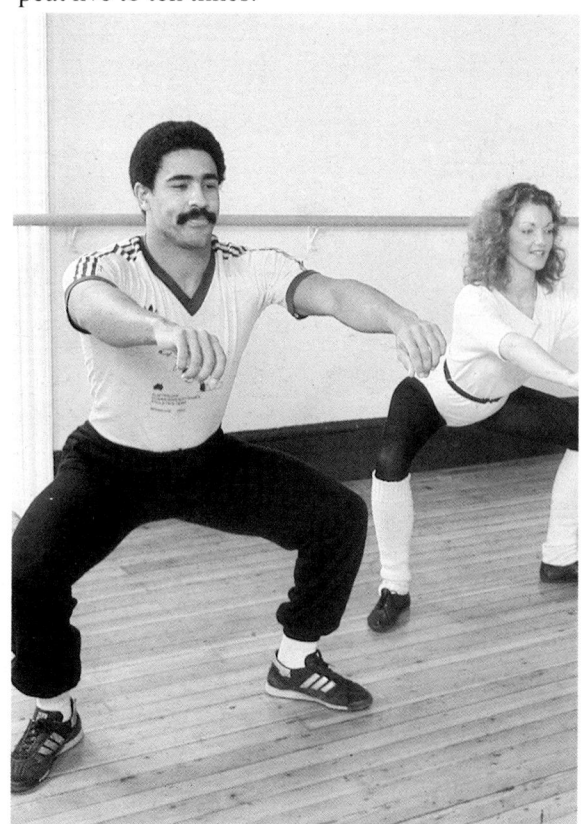

9 Bottoms down!

6 Kneel up, stretch out your left leg and lean over on your right hand. Now swing your left arm above your head and reach over as far as you can, keeping your body straight. Bounce twice, then lower your arm and repeat. Repeat the whole movement ten times, swap sides and repeat again. Concentrate on a good swing up and over with this one.

7 Stand up now, and get ready for some swinging movements. First, lean your hips to the right and step to the left, thrusting your arms to the left at the same time. Put your weight on your right foot, swing arms to the front, and close your right foot to your left. Repeat ten times.

8 Now do the same movement, this time leaning hips to the left, and stepping to the right. Repeat ten times, then alternate right and left swings for a further ten repeats. You must keep your back straight, head up and stomach and bottom tucked in while you perform this flowing dance step.

9 Now, feet wide apart, bend your knees, thrust your bottom back, arms forwards with palms down.

10 Now bring your pelvis forwards, shoulders back. Repeat back then forwards ten times.

11 Feet wide apart, back straight, arms straight out in front of you, bend forwards from the waist, keeping your head up. Do not arch that back.

12 Now lean forwards and touch the floor, head down. Bounce, two three, then raise your head. Down, two three, and up again.

13 Now stretch up and jump in the air, arms flung upwards, toes pointed. Repeat ten times.

This complete workout takes no longer than twenty minutes and exercises your whole body: stomach muscles (1, 2, 3); bottom (3); thighs (4); arms, torso, waist, midriff (5); hips, legs (6, 7); pelvis (8); back (9).

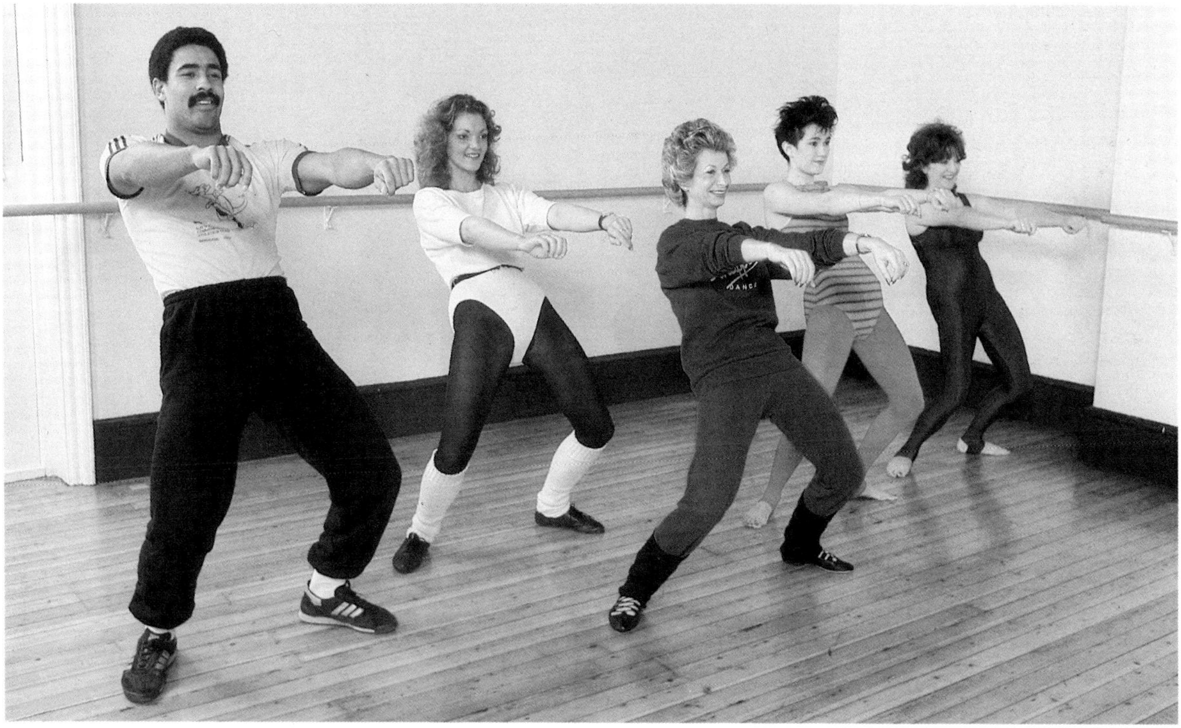

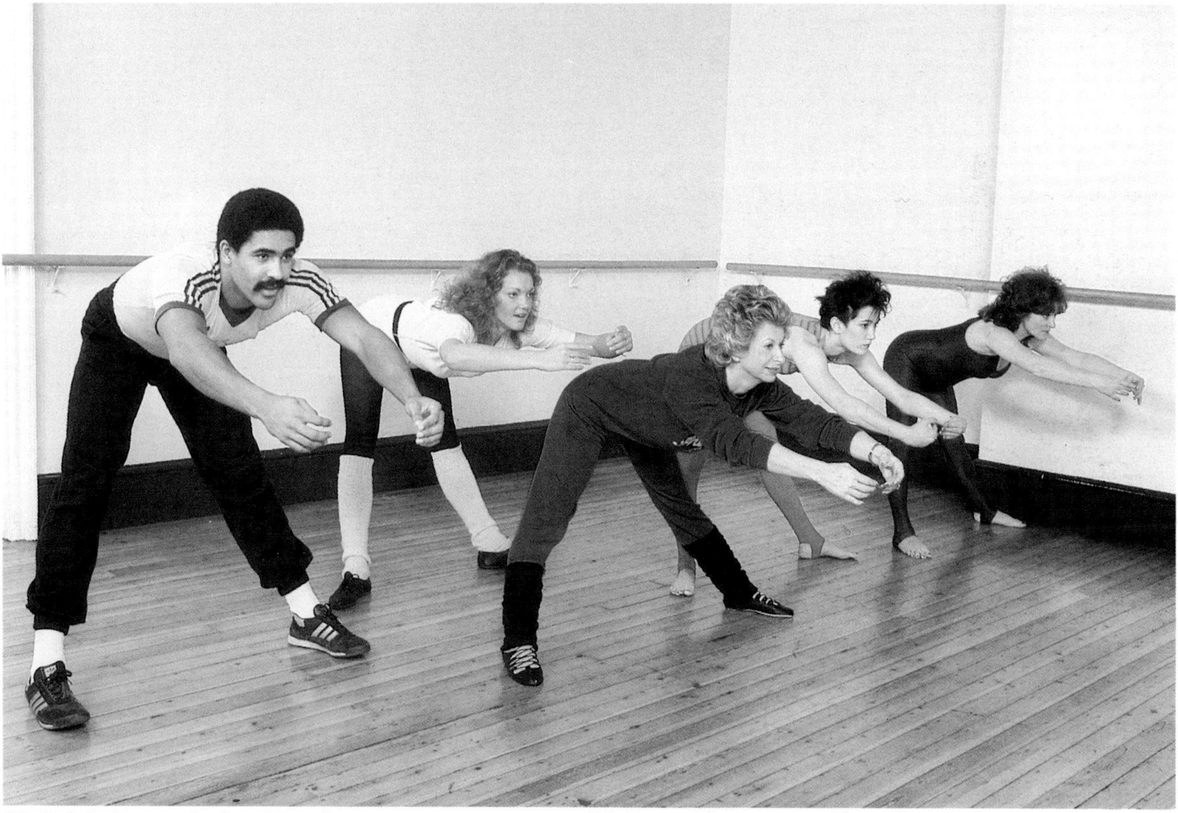

10 Pelvis forward, shoulders back　　　　　　*11 Feet wide apart and lean forward*

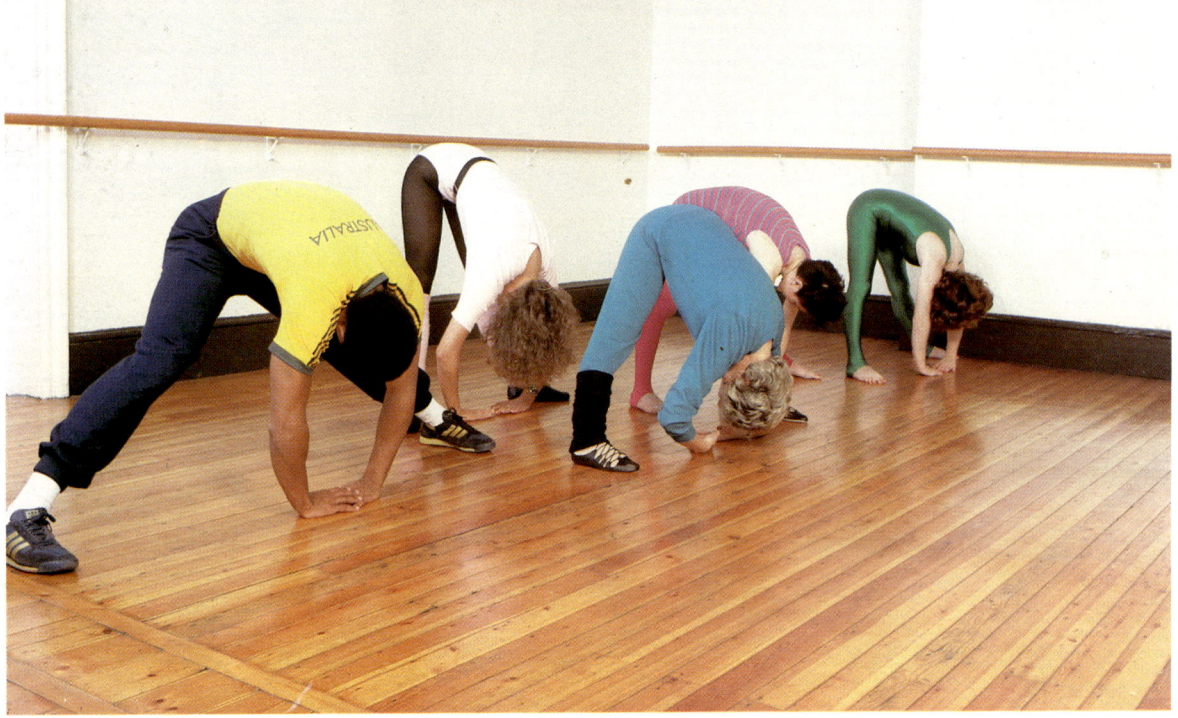

12 Legs wide apart, touch the floor

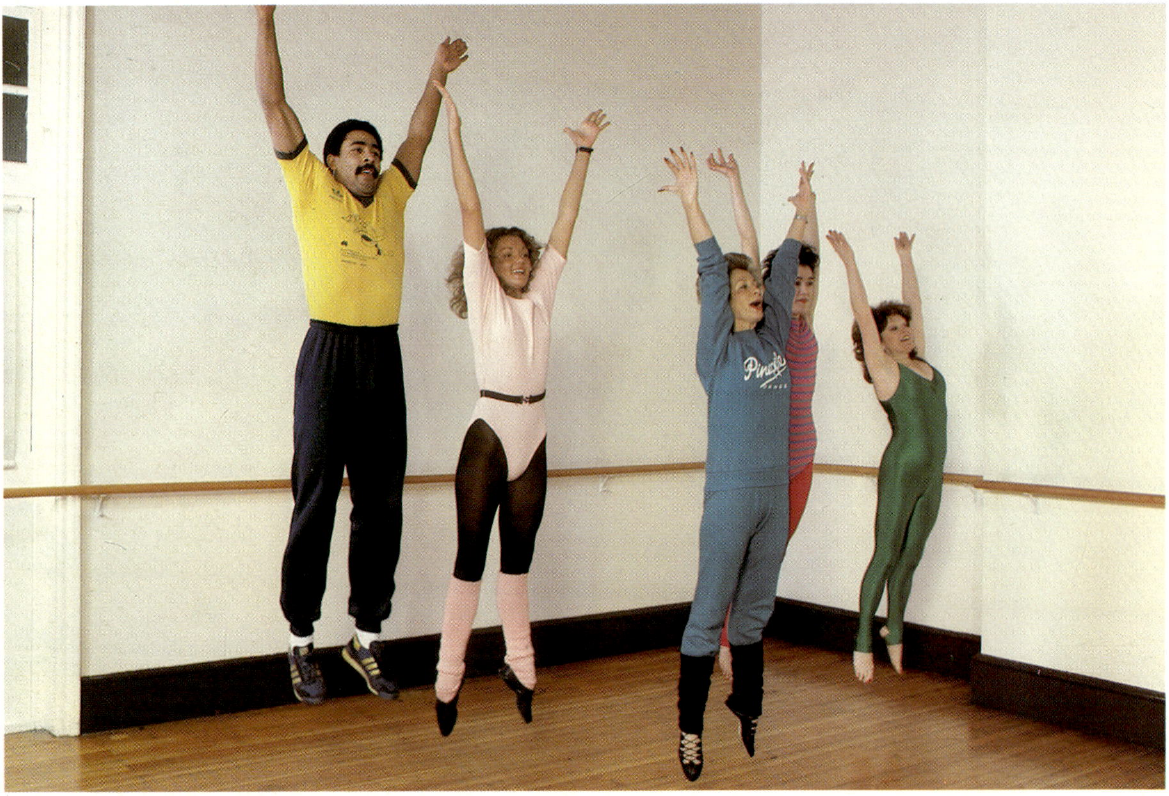

13 Stretch up and jump

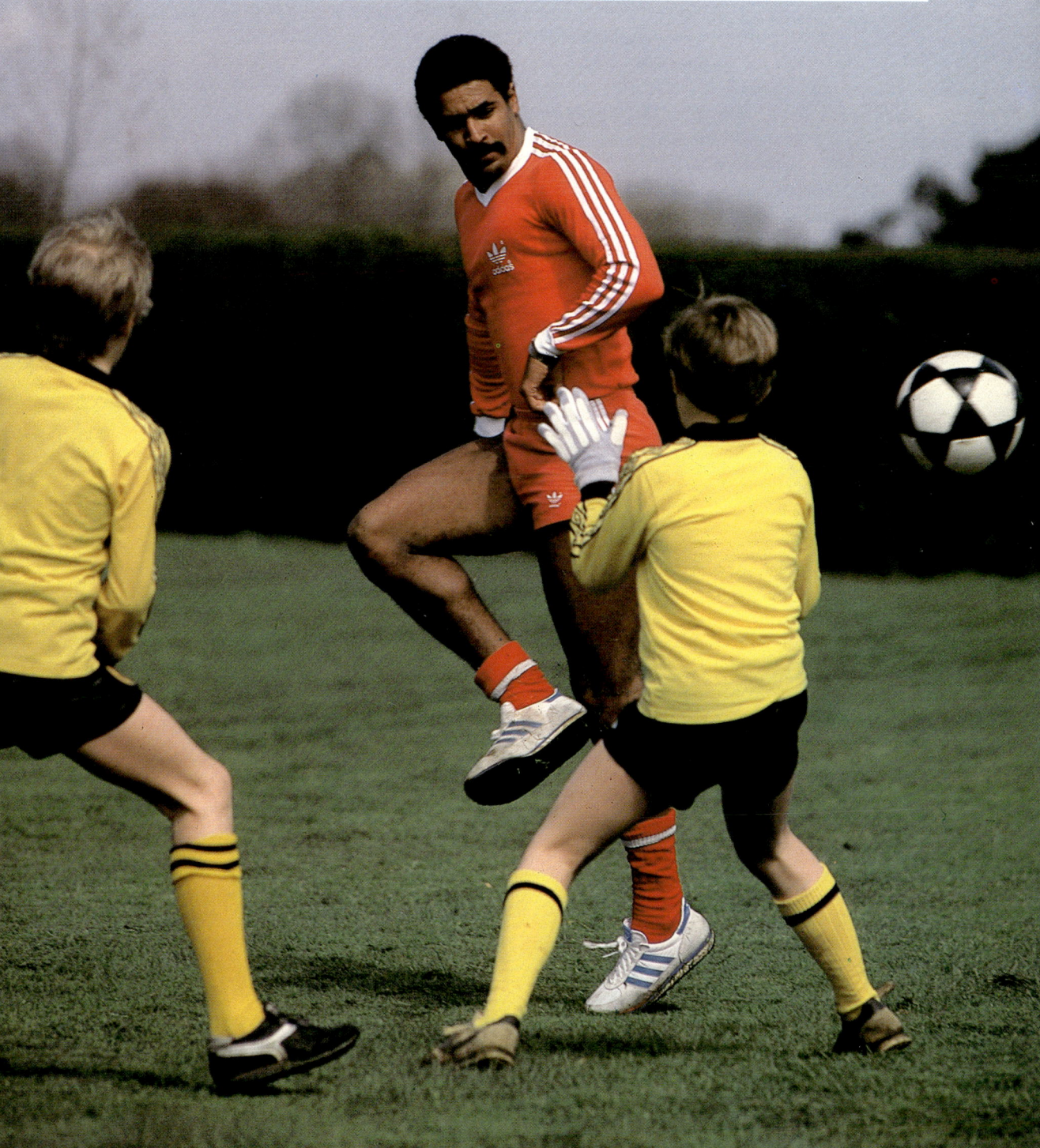

Chapter 11
Get fit for sport

Although I am a decathlete, I enjoy most other kinds of sport, too. For instance, we occasionally play basketball at Haringey when we are training. I also enjoy swimming, and all ball games, especially soccer. Soccer is my big game! I am really a frustrated footballer. I play anywhere up front – like any player I can kick with both feet! When I was younger I had trials for Fulham and Chelsea, and when I was fifteen, I used to play regularly with Fulham Juniors. Now, I play with Denis Waterman's Show Biz eleven! I usually try and turn out for the team every other week or so up until Christmas; after that I have to be careful not to get injured because the athletics season starts quite soon and it is risky for me to indulge in hazardous games, and the Show Biz team are a rough bunch! However, even when I am not playing, I am a keen soccer supporter. I support Ipswich Town because my brother Frank used to go to school up there, and we always went to the game when I visited him. I also admire Liverpool, because I once did a television programme called *Stopwatch* on BBC and spent a couple of days with the boys, and they made me really welcome.

Lots of youngsters ask me about specialising in one sport or another. Personally, I think that if you are a youngster who is a good all-rounder, you should continue like that. Let your body develop until you are eighteen or nineteen, and *then* decide how you want to specialise. You should not decide until the last possible moment because you are only closing other avenues which may turn out better for you. Similarly, it is a big mistake for parents and teachers to push a child into one particular field too soon. I believe you should encourage children by making training fun. Never make children do boring, repetitive exercises or things like twenty press-ups – they will be fed up in no time. Adults, too, are more likely to stick with a sport if they have a lot of fun with it. I have been lucky because no one has ever pushed me into sport or made it seem like a chore. People have always assumed that I am enjoying myself, which is true, most of the time.

I train for my own particular event in various ways, according to the skill required – and I feel certain that this thinking should be applied to all sports. There is no point in doing press-ups for hours if you are a footballer who is going to need strong legs, or spending a long time doing sit-ups if you are a darts player. I think a lot of football clubs could spend their time better. For long jump, high jump,

sprint starts and pole vault (which all demand incredibly strong legs), I work on my leg muscles doing 'bounding' exercises wearing a weighted jacket to make it harder work. You simply jump with both feet together from a knees-bent position in a 'bounding' movement as far as you can. I aim to improve my distance considerably during the pre-competition run-up, and then discard the jacket and find out what my legs can really do without being hampered. I recommend this to build up leg strength for soccer, ball games of other kinds, and, of course, for distance running.

Here are some fitness exercises for various sports, starting, naturally, with my second love – soccer:

SOCCER

Leg strengthening exercises

1 Stand with your legs shoulders' width apart, hands behind your head. Now bend your knees and 'bound' using both feet, landing as far forward as you can. Repeat five times. You can use this exercise as the basis for games and competitions with a group, or your team, or do it alone in your garden to build up those all-important leg muscles.

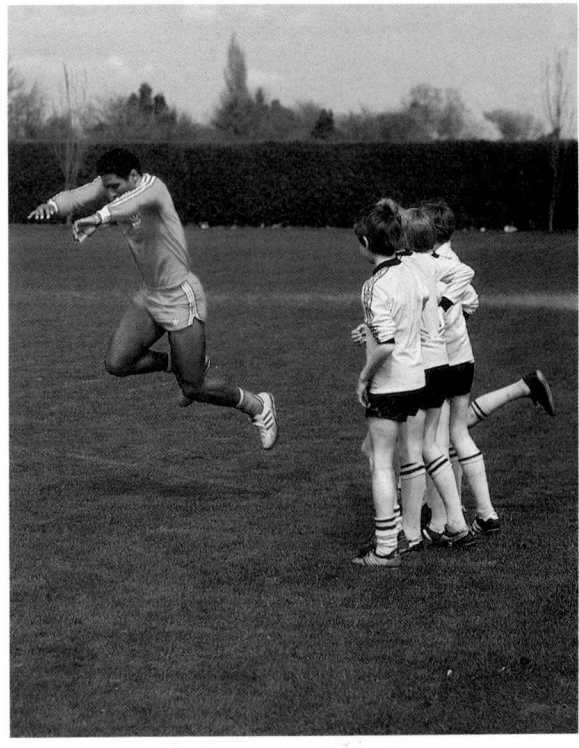

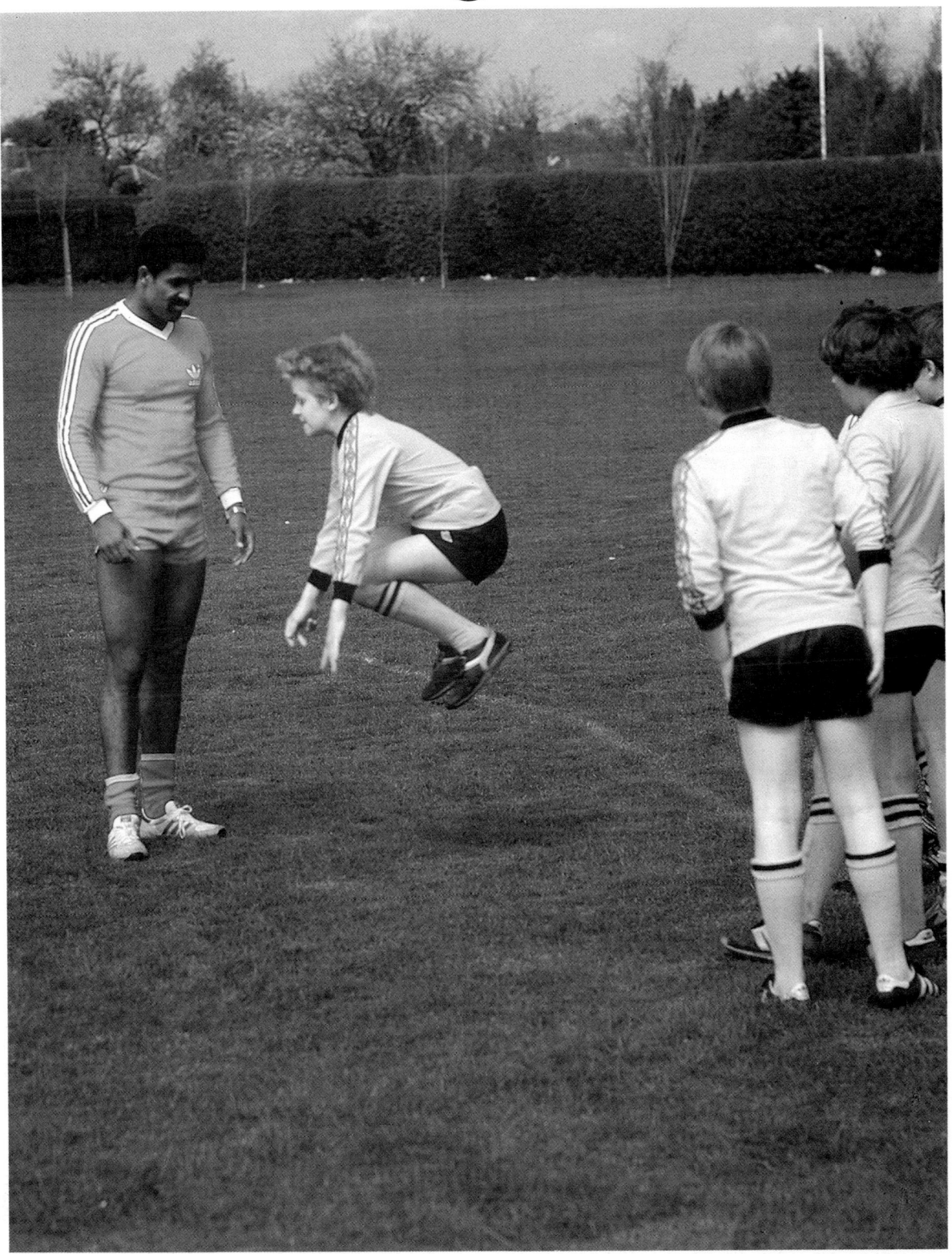

Bounding helps strengthen legs for soccer, long-jump, squash, tennis and many other sports. It is fun, too.

2 Stand facing a wall, stretch up and get someone to mark where your fingertips reach with a piece of chalk. Now take the chalk in your hand, leap as high as you can in the air, hand right above your head, and make another mark on the wall. Aim to improve your leap, lengthening the distance between the two marks. Like bounding, this gives legs super exercise. You can run a competition with this one as it does not matter if your friends are all different heights, since what counts is the distance *between* the marks.

3 Stand with feet apart, but parallel. Now press your legs strongly inwards, so that the feet roll in slightly and your inner thigh muscles tighten. Hold for a count of six, relax, then repeat six times.

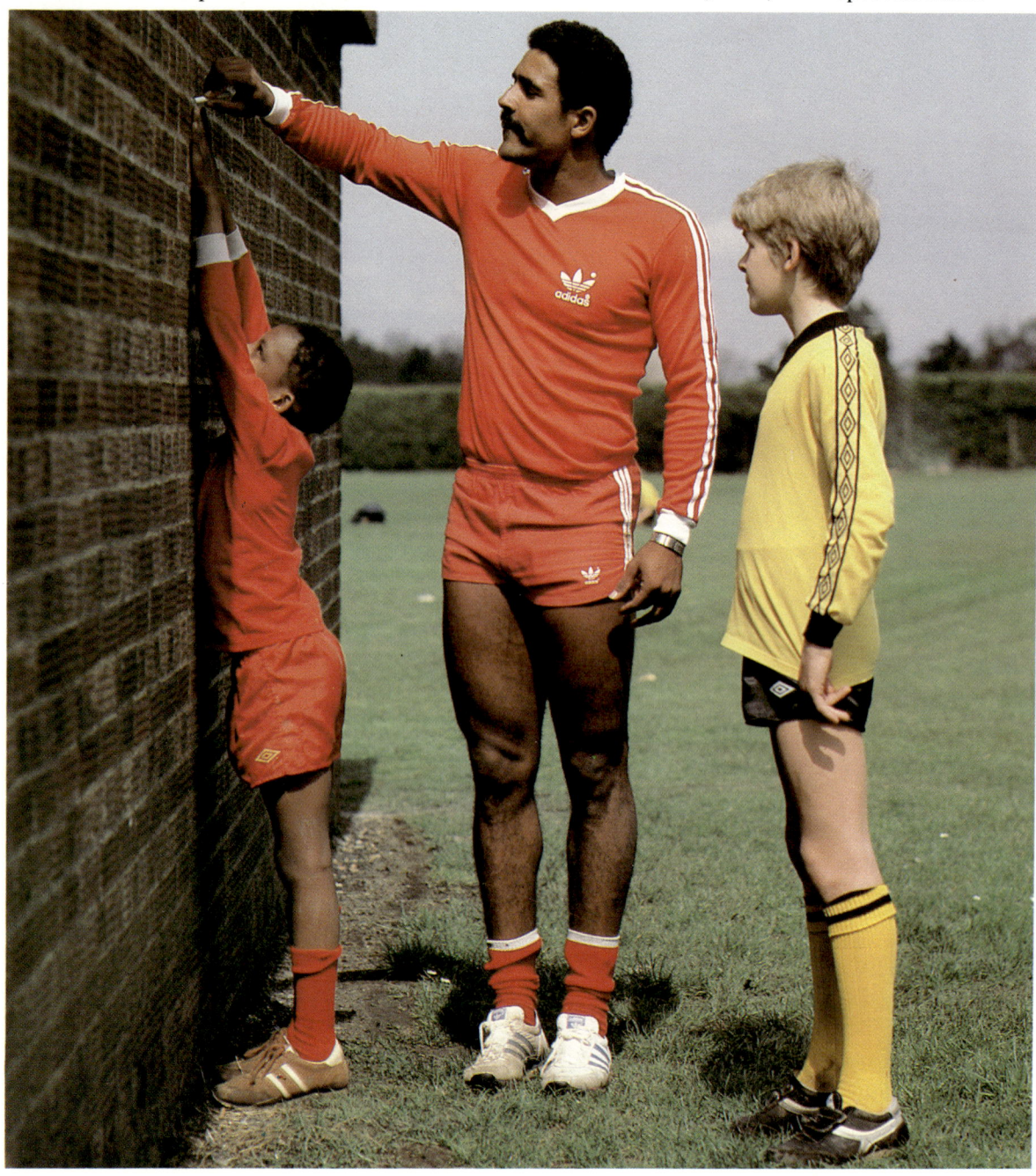

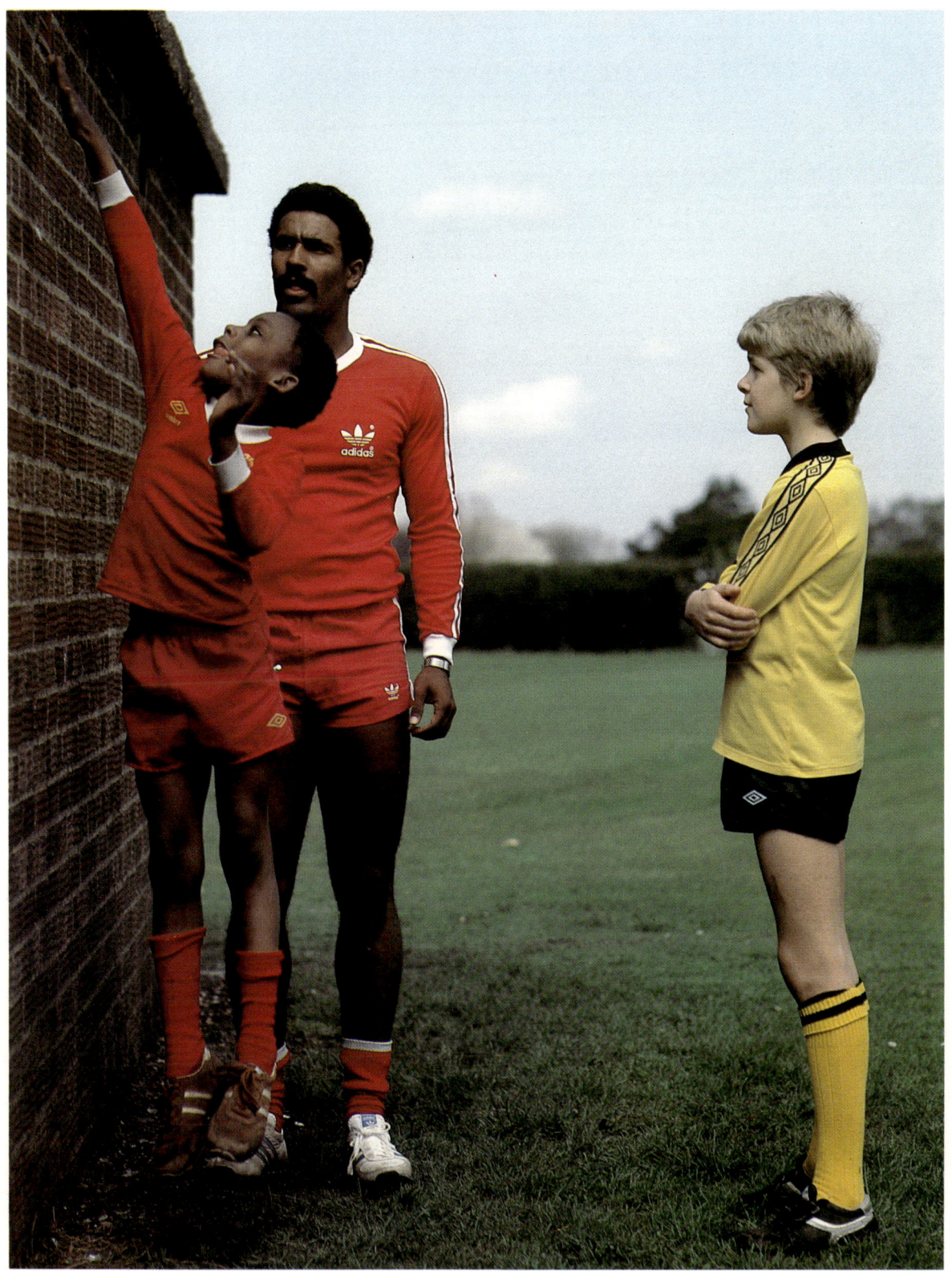

Skills

1 KICKING

Work in threes, one in the middle, two each side in a triangular pattern. Now play the ball first to the man in the middle, let him return, then kick to the far man who repeats the pattern. Vary your kicks, using inside and toe, moving back, sideways, dummying, and feinting. This is much more interesting than simply working in twos.

Now mark targets on a wall and shoot at them, returning the rebounds first time and working with a partner for alternate shots.

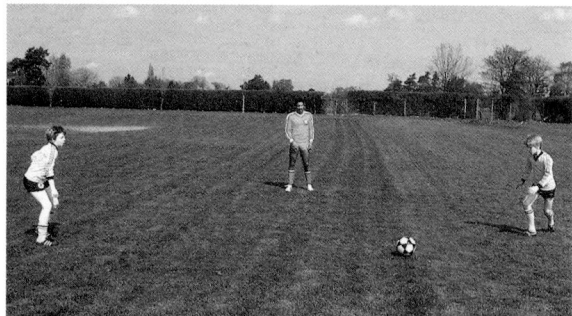

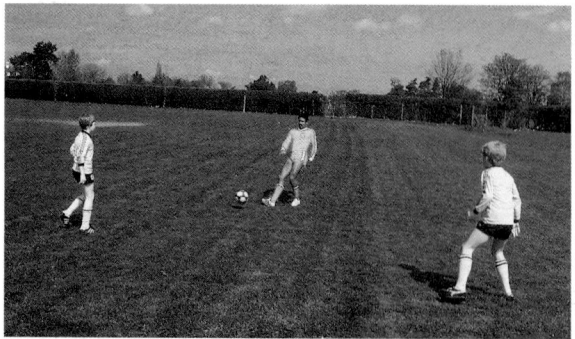

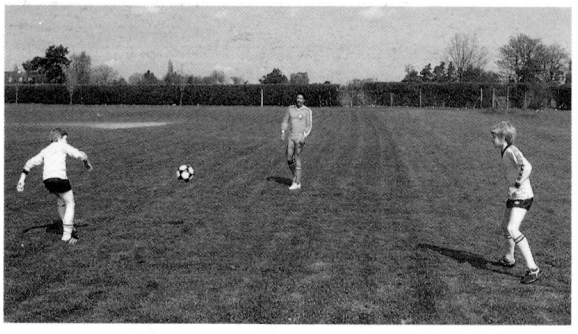

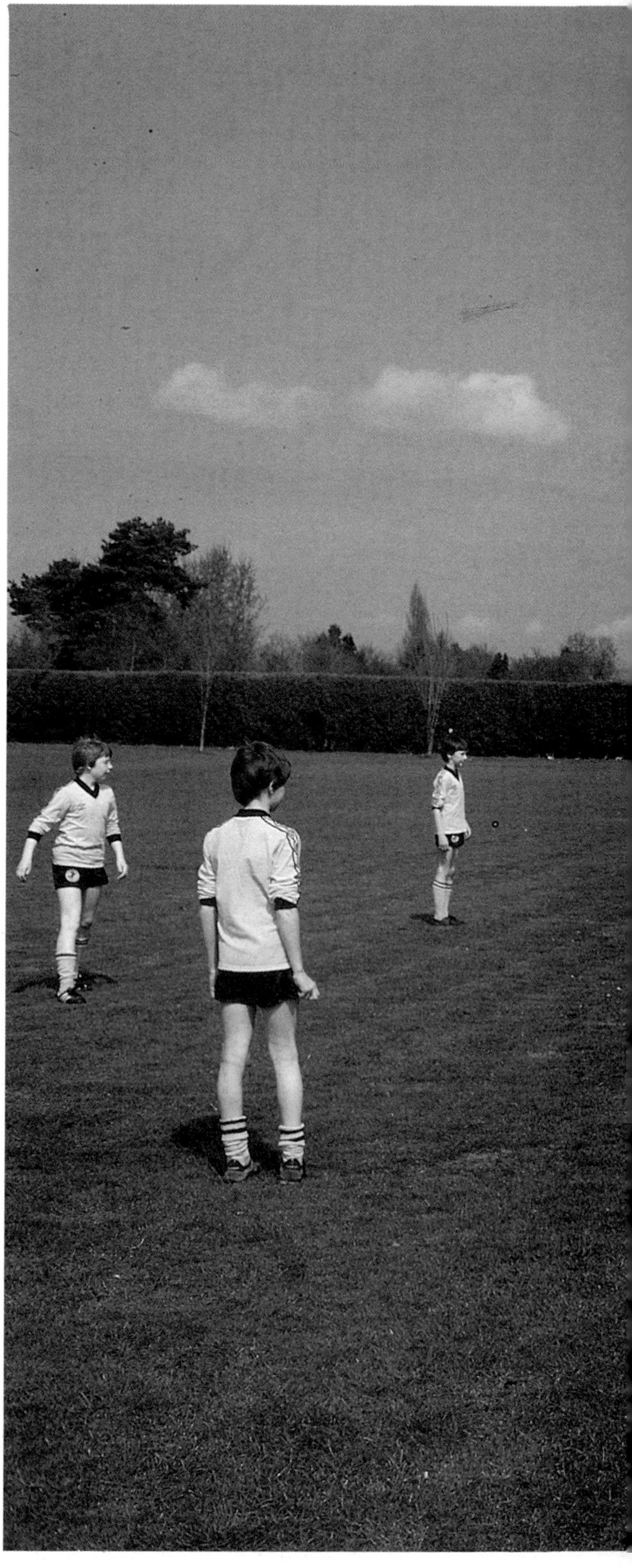

Ball control is vital – learn to use both feet, like me!

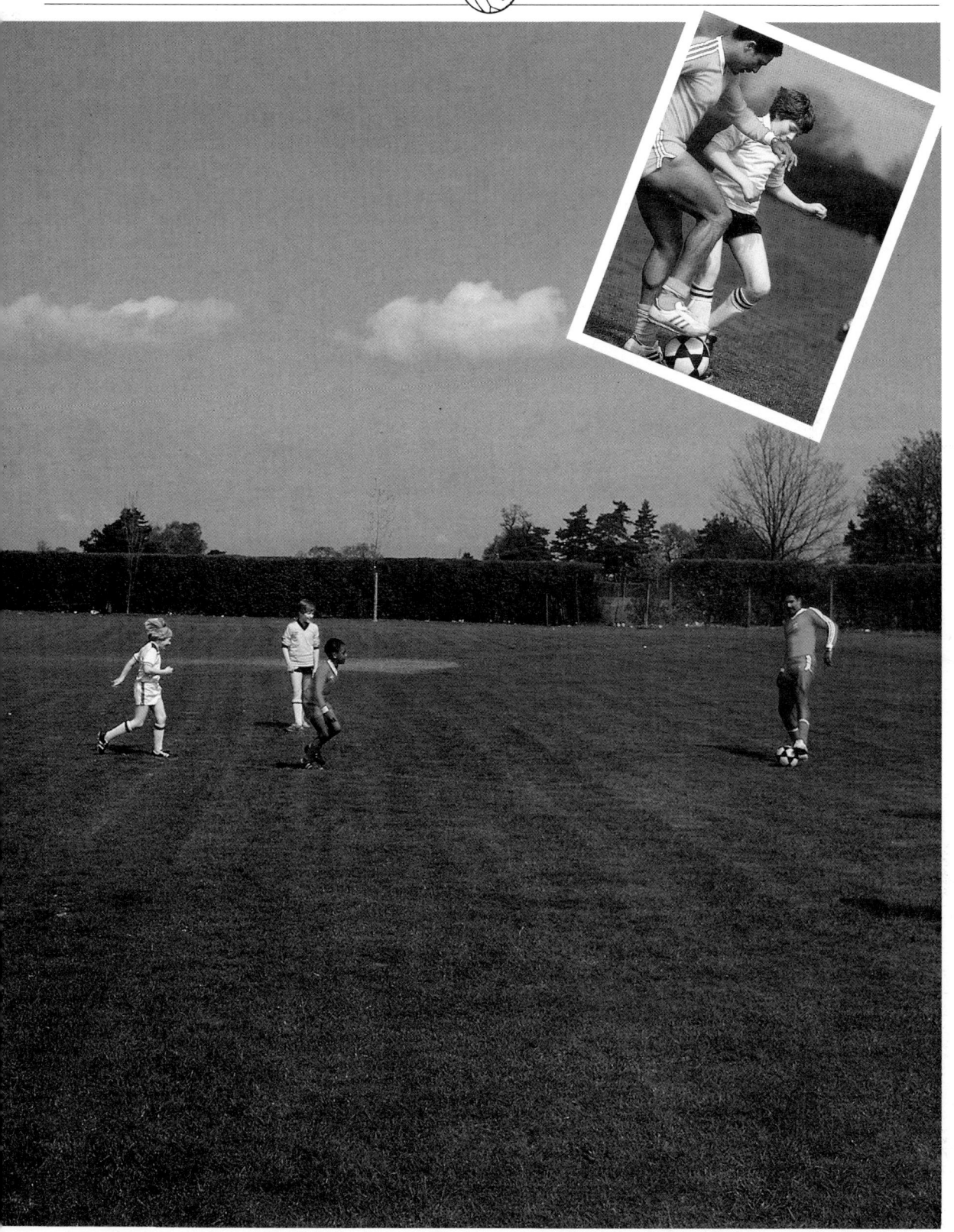

2 HEADING

Play 'head tennis', with four or five players each side of the net or rope. You may play the ball with the feet or the head, but you must head it *over* the net. Each dropped ball is one point against your team.

3 BALL CONTROL

Play 'pig in the middle'. Six players pass the ball round a circle. Two players in the middle make a real effort to win the ball. Players take it in turns to go into the middle.

4 GOAL KEEPING

Stand with your back to the pitch on the goal line. Get a mate to shoot at you, yelling when he makes contact with the ball. You must turn quickly and deal with the shot.

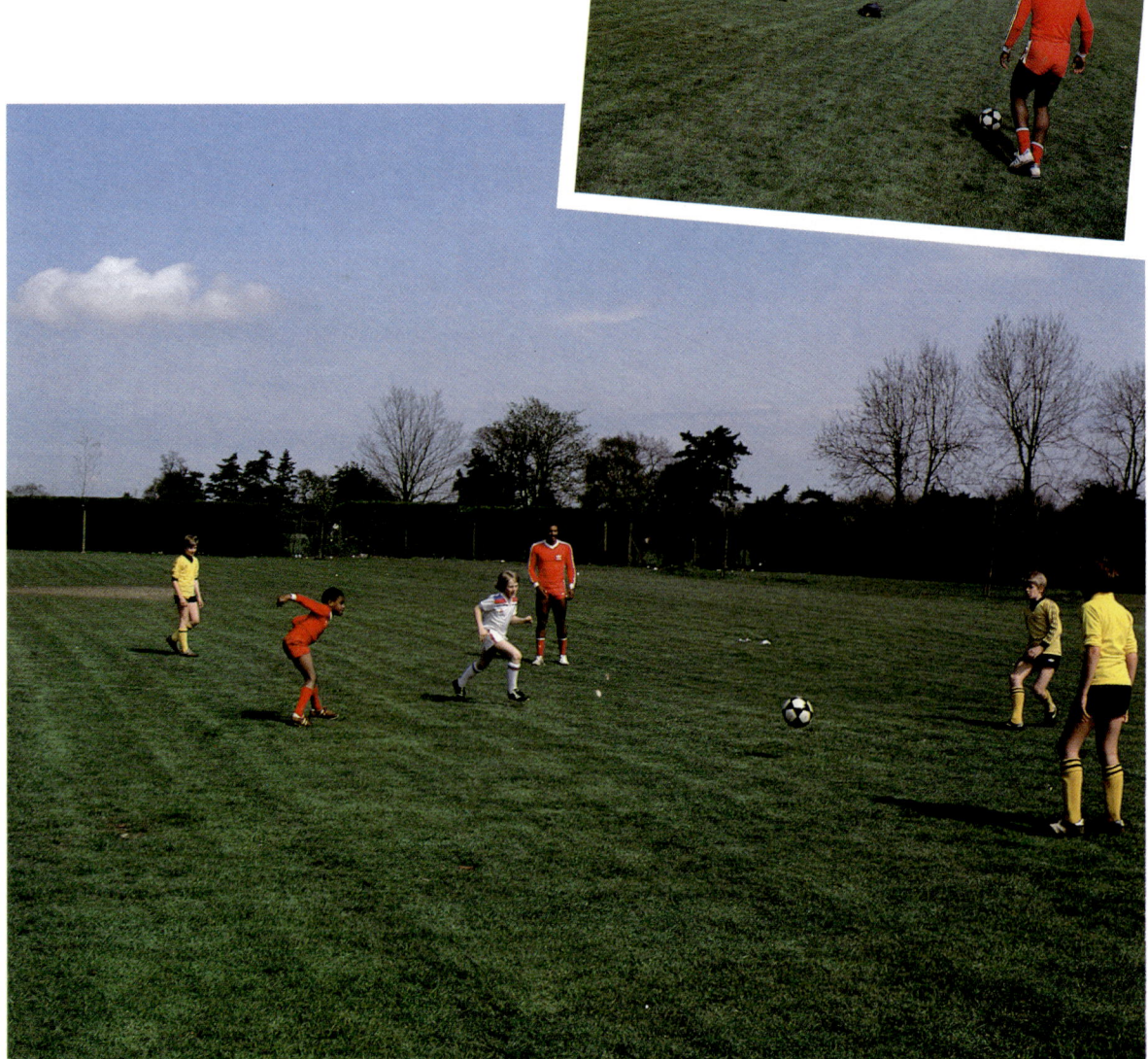

Play 'pig in the middle' and get some excellent tackling practice

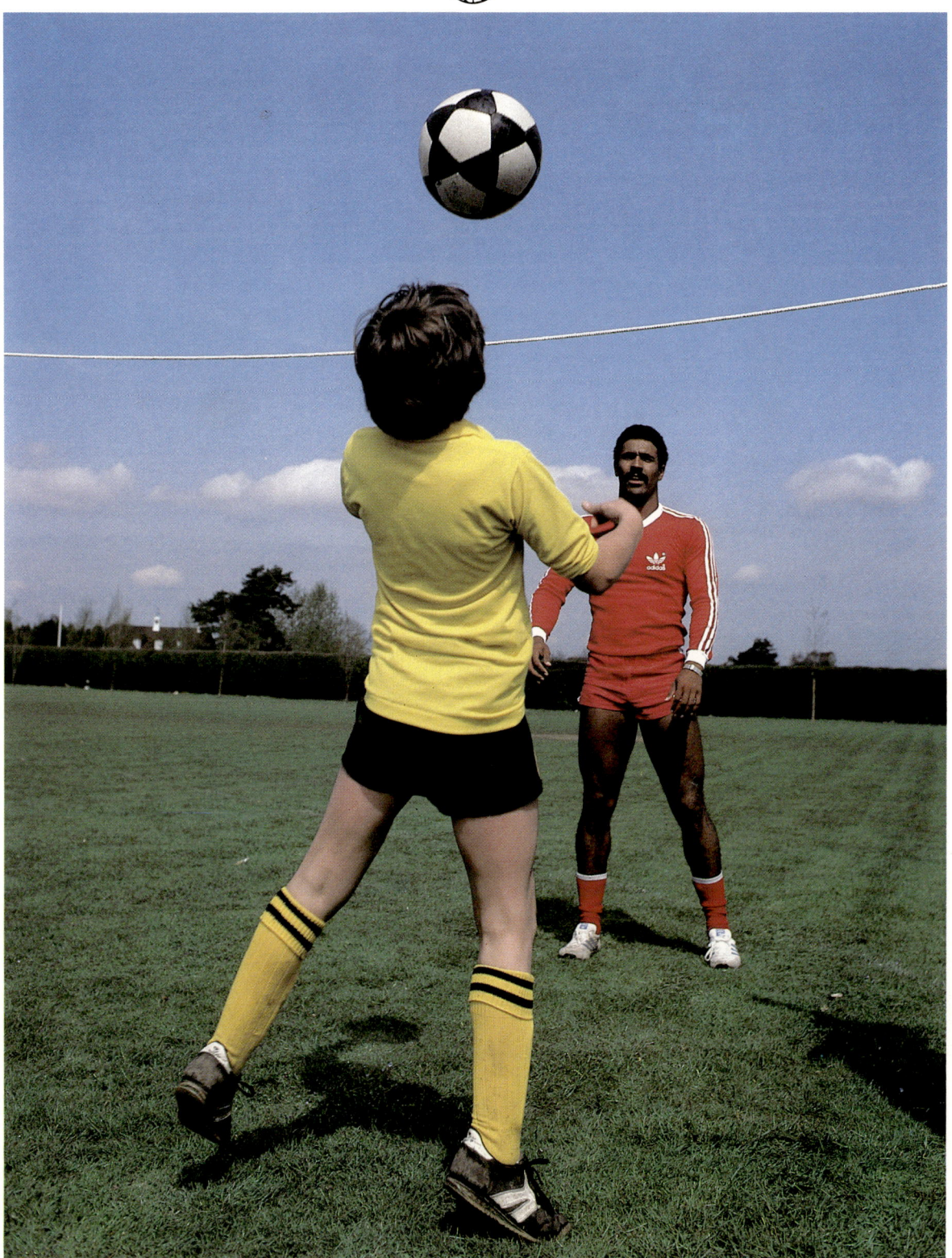

Head tennis is a good way to develop one of the vital soccer skills

TENNIS AND SQUASH

Tennis is very much a game of psychological strength as well as physical fitness. The great players use all their mental skills – and sometimes reveal much more about the innermost workings of their psyche than they realise. In squash, too, sheer mental determination is almost as important as ability, and the power which is released on the court is almost tangible. In both games, concentration is of paramount importance. I think it is a good idea to work on this aspect with a programme of deep breathing and yoga-type exercises, then work on speed and strength.

Breathing

Stand straight, hands over your ribcage. Now breathe in deeply, feeling your ribs rise and visualising your body as a container for all that air – it is being filled up like a balloon. Now, breathe out, slowly, with great control, imagining the fatigue and tension passing out of your body as you do so. Keep it up for a few moments, aiming to make the breathing-in last as long as the breathing-out part. On court, use this breathing technique between hard-fought rallies to give you extra powers of recovery and energy for the next shot.

Shuttle sprinting

Place three balls in a line at the other end of the garden or about twenty-five yards away in the park. Now, with a friend timing you or timing yourself, run to pick up one ball, bring it back to the starting point, then get the next, until all three are back. Aim to improve your time over the same distance.

Chinning

Grasp a branch of a tree or a bar in the gym and hang from both arms, feet off the ground. Now use your arms to pull yourself up so that your chin reaches the spot just above the branch. This is great fun, and also good for arm strength for those powerful shots.

Trunk rotation

Stand feet apart, holding your racquet behind your head with both hands. Rotate your trunk as far as possible to the right, then to the left, keeping your heels on the ground. Repeat complete movement ten times. This is good for ensuring mobility in the trunk when you have to twist and turn to cope with awkward shots.

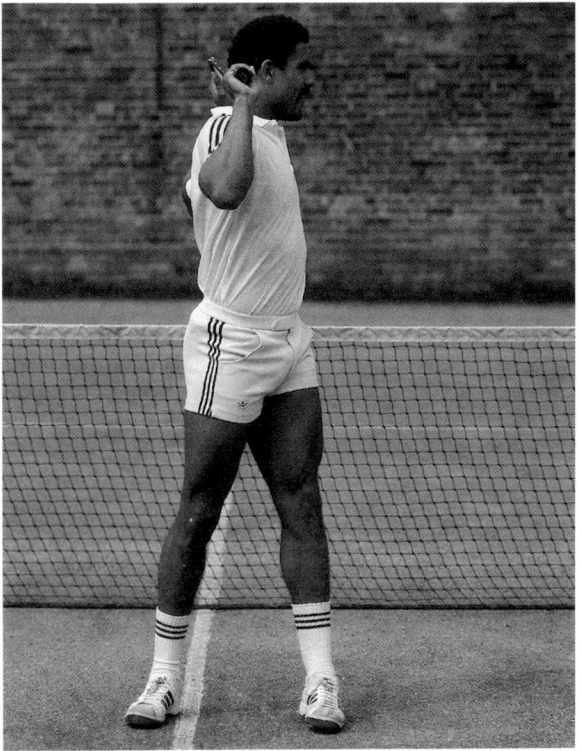

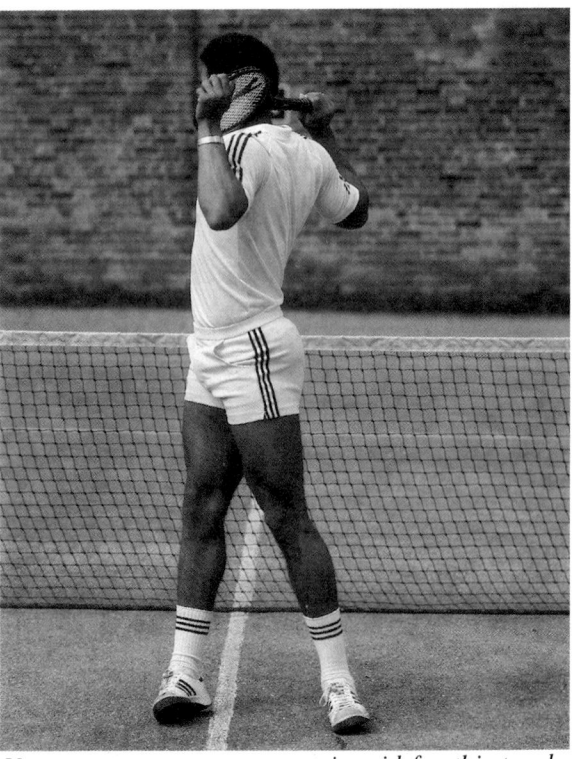

Use your racquet as an exercise aid for this trunk-twisting movement

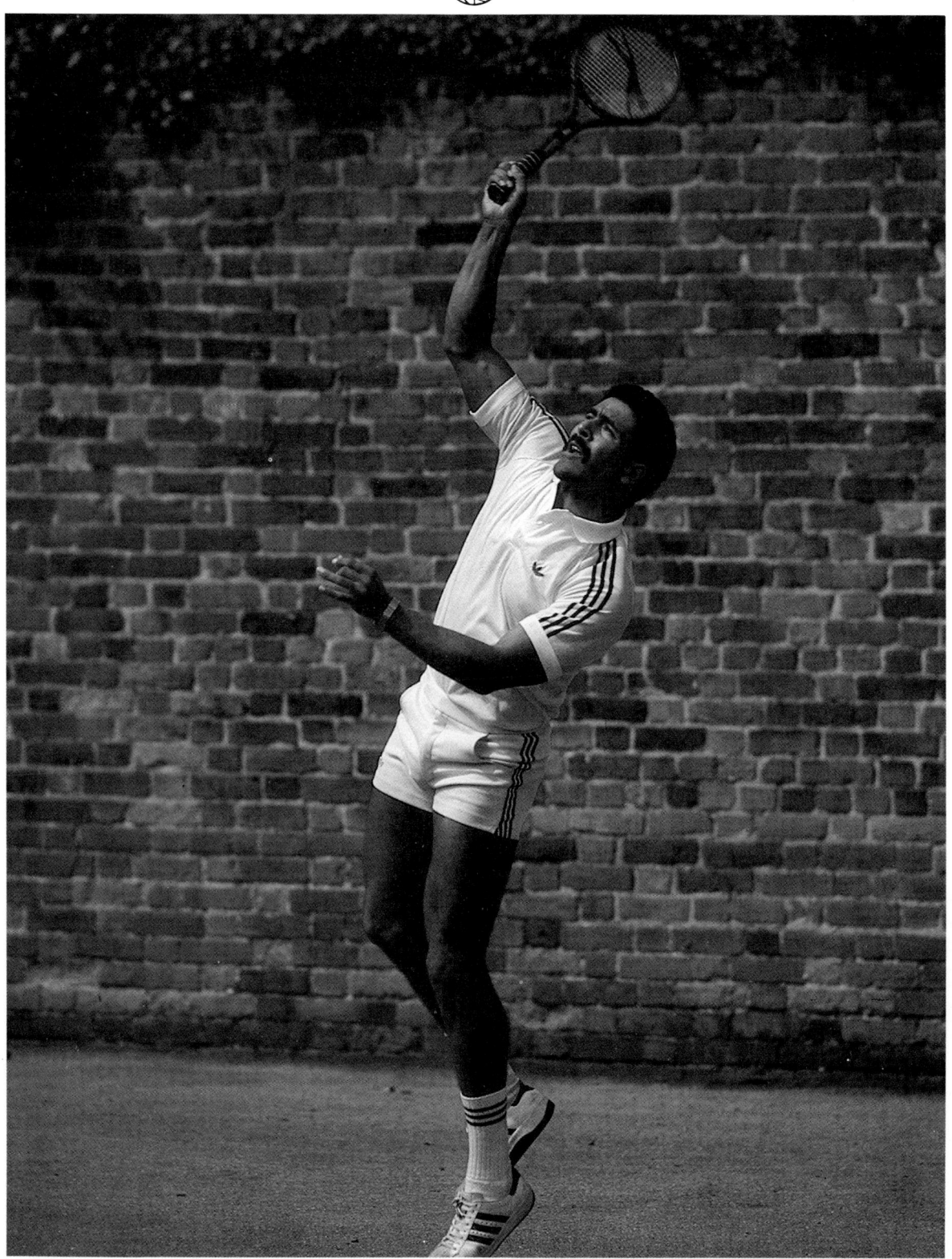

Many games are won or lost on service. That is why I am practising!

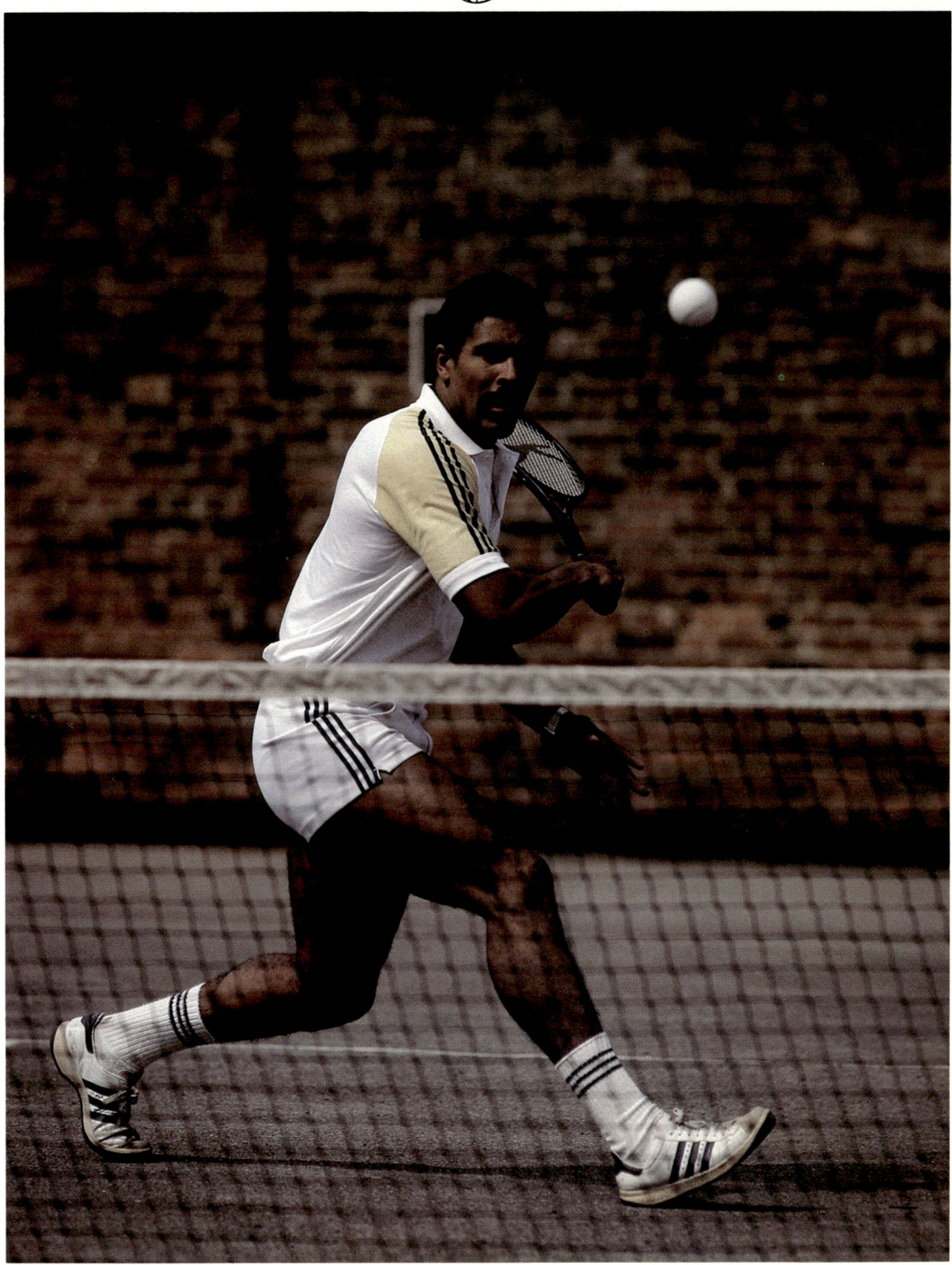

Backhand weak? Work at it!

GOLF

Legs are more important in golf than you might think – stance is a vitally important part of your swing preparation, and control over the centre part of your body will give you much more control over the way you hit the ball. Sloppy swingers often need more leg and hip control than wrist or arm strength. These exercises cover all four:

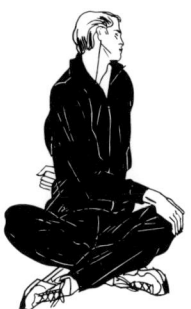

Twisting

Sit cross-legged on the floor, back straight. Now place your right hand on your left knee, your left hand behind you. Turn your head and chest as far round to the left as possible keeping your spine erect. Hold for a count of three, return to the front, then repeat to the right. Repeat the whole movement six times.

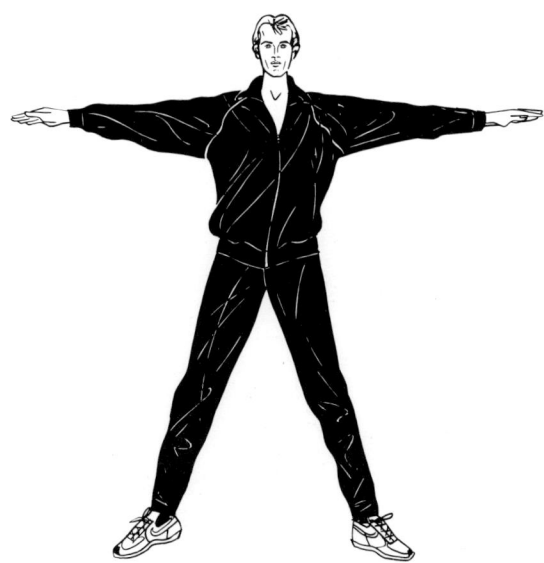

Side-pushing

Stand with feet wide apart, arms outstretched, palms down. Now push your shoulders to the left, stretching out the left arm. Return to starting position, push shoulders to the right. Repeat ten times each side. You must keep your back straight and legs firm throughout the exercise.

Wrist joint

Sit or stand comfortably, arms straight out in front of you. Rotate the hands, left, then right, then push fingertips up, then down. Keep it up for a minute or so.

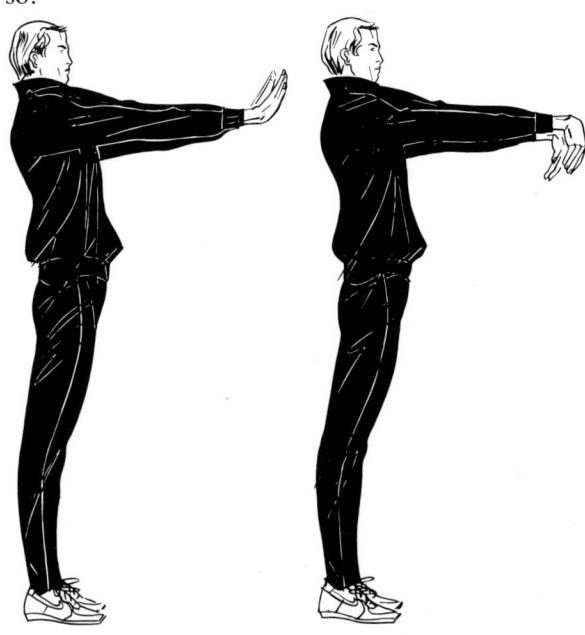

Shoulder rotation exercise

Sit comfortably, legs apart, feet flat on the floor. Now lift your arms to shoulder level, bending them up to form a right angle and pressing backwards.

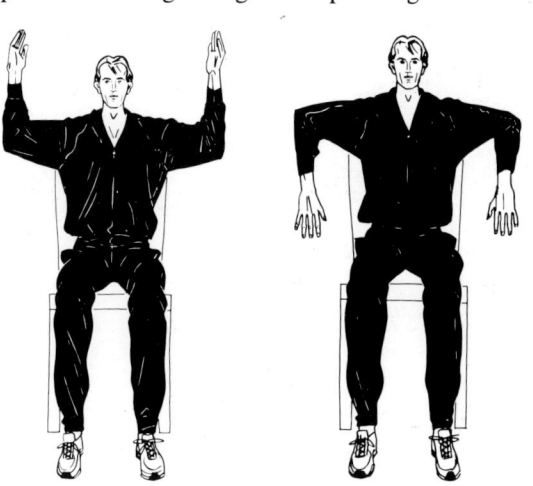

Keep the upper arms raised at shoulder level as you turn your forearms so that the fingers point downwards, holding the right angle at the elbow. Press backwards and downwards for a count of three. Then relax. Repeat three times.

DARTS

No, throwing the javelin is *not* just a glorified version of darts playing – we are always told by our coaches that the *last* thing we must do is imagine that we are holding a giant dart! The very best exercise for darts is to play the game as often as possible, but it can also help to do wrist-strengthening exercises and eye relaxing movements to rest tired eyes.

Wrists

Sit at a table or bench with elbows on the table, hands pressed together in a 'praying' position. Now push hands down, away from your body. Hold the position for a count of six, then raise them. Repeat ten times. Now 'throw' your hands away from you, keeping your elbows tucked against your body, forearms and wrists still. Repeat fifteen to twenty times.

Eyes

Sit with hands in your lap, feet comfortable, back straight. Look straight ahead, then left, right, up and down. Now focus on something in the middle distance – a picture on the wall, for instance (A). Focus on something in the far distance – a tree in the garden which you can see through the window is a suitable object (B). Rapidly switch from object A, to object B, ten times.

SKI-ING, WINDSURFING

Continental and American ski-ing and windsurfing instructors moan about the British and their wobbly legs and bad sense of balance. I think we are bad at first because snow ski-ing is not a traditional sport in this country, although it is becoming more popular. We are not used to sports which demand grace and co-ordination in quite the way that these skills do, although our own soccer does have a certain balletic

quality at times! Before you go on a ski-ing holiday (on snow or water), or decide to go off windsurfing, do try these exercises for the relevant parts of the body:

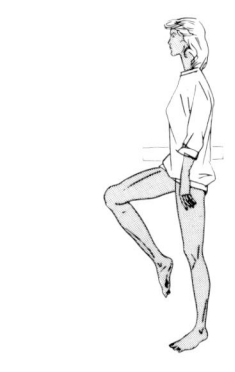

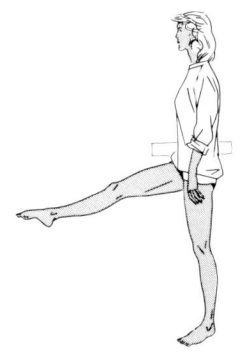

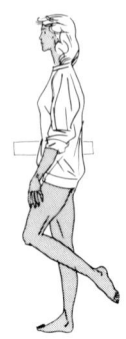

For knees, thighs

Stand sideways to a chair, using the back of the chair for balance, arm straight. Now bend your right knee, raise it, stretch the leg out, lower it. Repeat with left knee and leg. Repeat whole movement with alternate legs, ten times. Now make large circles with the foot of your outside leg, just off the ground, clockwise, then anti-clockwise. Change sides and repeat once.

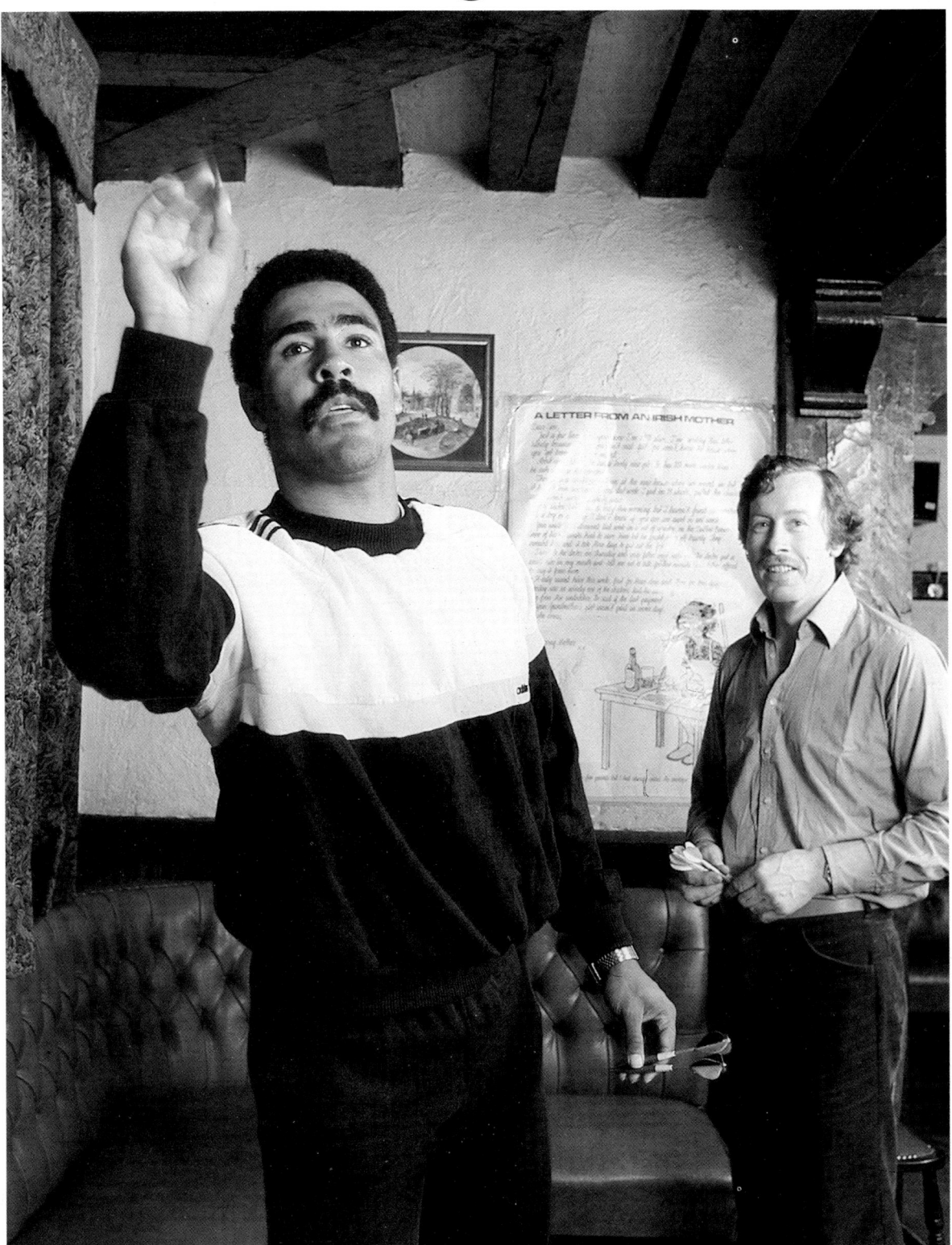

Bullseye! Get your eye in for darts with the exercise opposite!

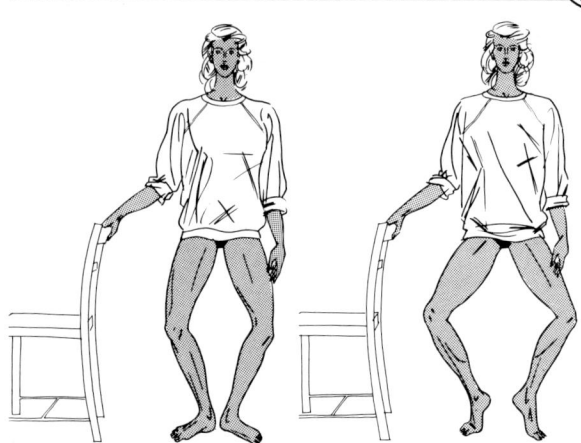

on the chair seat, feet together, knees slightly bent. Relax your shoulders, pull in your stomach. Now lift your right leg, cross it over your left leg to get as close as you can to the floor the other side, keeping shoulders on the ground. Raise it again, go back to starting position and repeat with left leg. Repeat five times.

For hips, pelvic girdle

Still using the chair, place heels together and bend your knees as low as you can. Raise up on your toes. Keep your back straight and do not wobble throughout the exercise. Repeat five times.

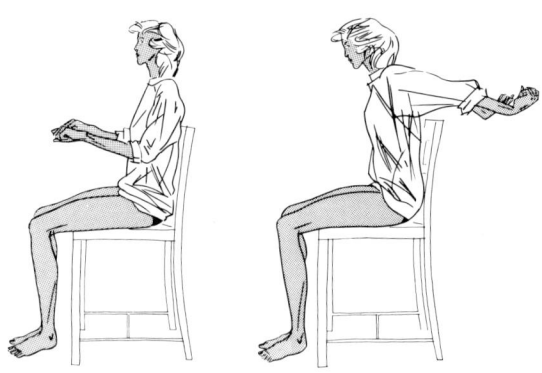

For upper arms

Sit comfortably, arms bent forward, hands in loose fists, palms down. Straighten the arms backwards, punching them as far back as possible. Repeat five to ten times.

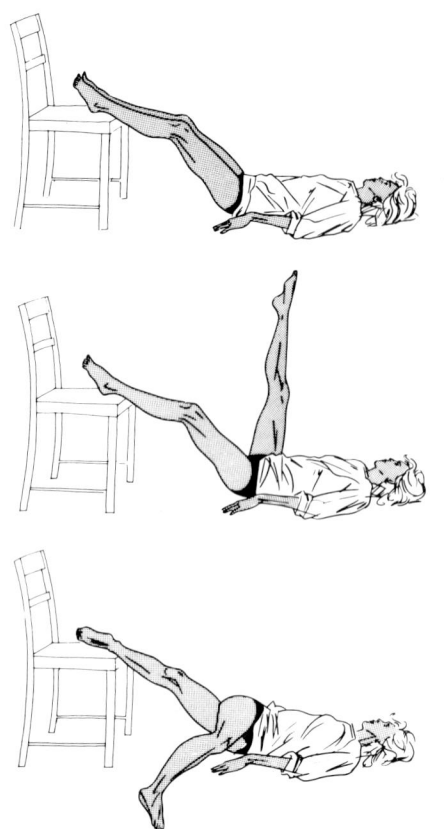

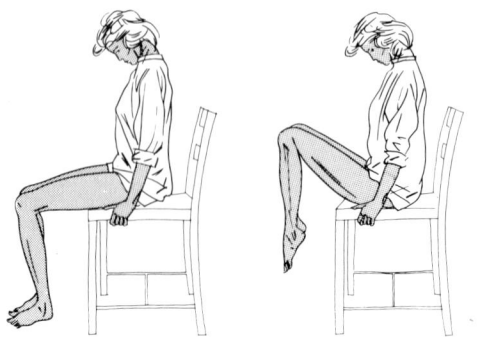

For stomach muscles

Sit on that chair this time, knees bent, feet together. Hold the *seat* of the chair with both hands. Drop your head, resting your chin on your chest. Lift your knees and point your toes, keeping your back perfectly straight. Hold for a count of two, then lower feet, raise head. You must breathe out, pulling in your stomach as you raise your knees, breathe in as you lower them. Repeat five to ten times.

For legs, hips

Lie on your back on the floor with your legs resting

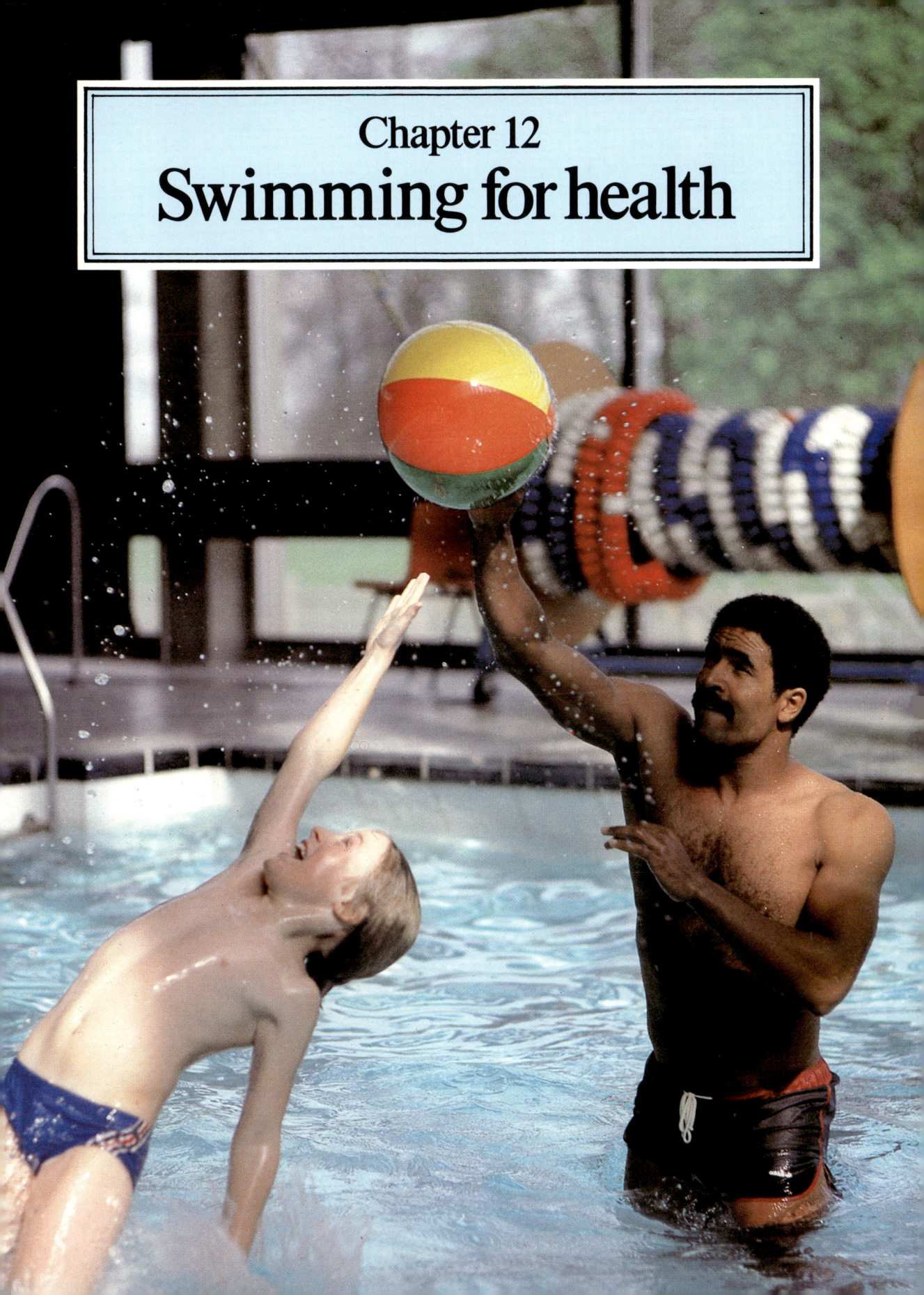

I first learnt to swim when I was seven years old. I was on a boating holiday at the time, travelling from London to Birmingham by canal. There were other children on the trip and they could all swim; they would dive off the boat with confidence while I had to cling on. I watched for a while from the boat, and then decided to learn. By the end of the holiday, I was diving with confidence, too. Ever since, I have been keen on swimming – it is a good form of exercise for all parts of the body, and it is a fun way to relax. I usually go swimming in the summer with a crowd – it makes a break from intensive training and yet I do not feel too guilty because I know I am getting a workout as well as a 'rest'. We usually swim a few lengths and then play some games – walking races backwards through the pool are one favourite, and we sometimes play a form of water-polo, which ends up with a lot of splashing!

Which all sounds like fun and games – but is actually doing us some good. Water is the ideal medium for exercise, especially if you are tense or tired, or are recovering from illness or injury. 'Hydrotherapy', as water exercises are called, has been used to aid recovery since Roman times, and is a highly important treatment for patients with muscular problems, the handicapped and elderly. Water works to help you exercise in two important ways. First, its resistance (the pressure against your body) helps to build up strength – you have to exert muscles to get through the water. Second, its buoyancy supports the weight of your body, relieving the pressure of gravity on your spine, and allowing the muscles of the legs and back, which usually have to work very hard to keep you standing up, to relax for a change.

Movements in the water therefore involve less tension, there is less build-up of waste-products in the blood stream, so that you never feel stiff and leaden after swimming. Even if you cannot swim, you can use these properties to your advantage in your keep-fit campaign: you can do simple water exercises, play games, and generally relax in the water (or in your own bath at home), and you can use hydrotherapy on holiday: just lying at the water's edge letting the waves wash over your body is a form of 'exercise', which is excellent for your circulation and helps you relax. And if you have back, knee, hip, ankle or general tension problems, there is no doubt that water works wonders.

Here are some exercises to try out in your local pool which will do great things for your body and your mental health. They are good for children to try, too. You do not have to be able to swim to do them and they will help build up your confidence if you cannot quite manage to take that first reluctant leap into the deep water! Many older people I meet never had the chance to learn to swim when they were younger – there just were not the facilities in those days – but they find that they can learn quite quickly with a little bit of instruction. Most pools have instructors who are only too willing to help you, and once you are confident, swimming really is one of the cheapest, most beneficial sports of all.

Warm up by doing a few jumps, holding on to the side if you like. Have a good splash about for a while to get your circulation going and relax your muscles.

1 *For neck, spine, waist, arms*

Now turn sideways on to the side of the pool, hold the edge, arm bent so that you are standing very close to it. Turn your head to the right, stretch your right arm out. Lean out, straightening your arm, keeping your feet close to the pool. You will not fall over! Now stretch your right arm up and over your head, leaning inwards towards the pool. Do five each side.

2 *For hands, arms, calves, Achilles tendon*

Face the side of the pool at a spot where water is at chest level. Now hold on to the rail with both hands, crouch up against the wall close to it, with your head tucked down. Now straighten your arms and legs, pushing away, and keeping your heels firmly against the side. Do not let go. Repeat five times.

3 *For spine, ankles, legs*

With the water at waist level or deeper, face the rail and hold it with both hands, about 90 cm (3′) apart. Now let your legs float up behind you, and kick, keeping knees straight, taking very small 'steps'. Do about ten, then turn over, and do another ten.

4 *For stomach, thighs, spine*

Stand in water to just above your waist. Now clasp your hands behind your head. Lift your left knee up, right elbow down (try to touch one with the other).

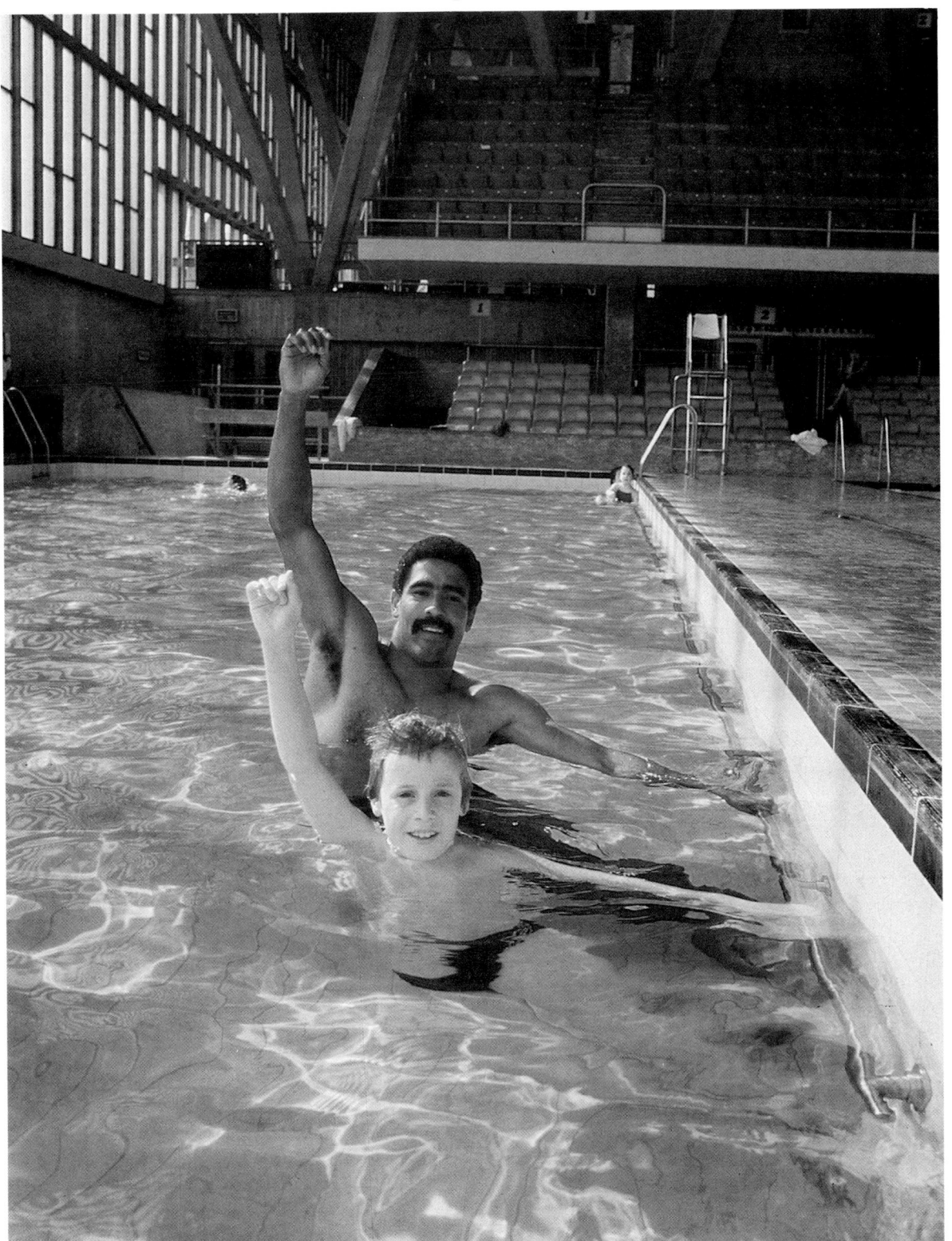

For neck, spine, waist, arms. You will not fall over doing this exercise because the water helps keep you steady.

Straighten up, and repeat with your right knee, left elbow. Repeat the whole movement five times.

5 *For waistline, ribcage, breathing*

Stand side-by-side in the water with a partner. Both open your legs as wide as possible, keeping your balance, and hold hands. Now raise the outside arms together and lean inwards to touch hands over your head, stretching really well from the waist. Straighten up, and repeat five times. You can do this one alone if you like, with one foot against the side of the pool for balance.

6 *For legs, posture, balance*

With water at waist-level, raise your hands straight out in front of you, palms down, and walk backwards through the water for a few steps. Walk forwards again, then backwards, then forwards. Try to keep your balance and posture perfect.

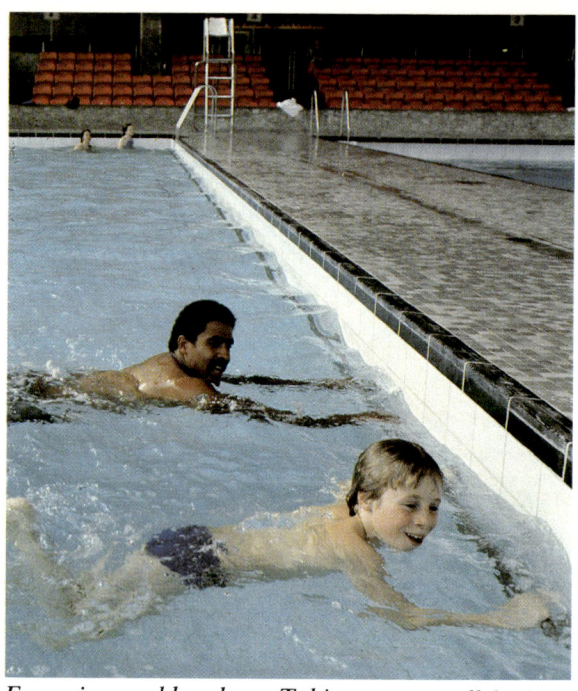

For spine, ankles, legs. Taking very small kicking 'paces' really does exercise those leg muscles.

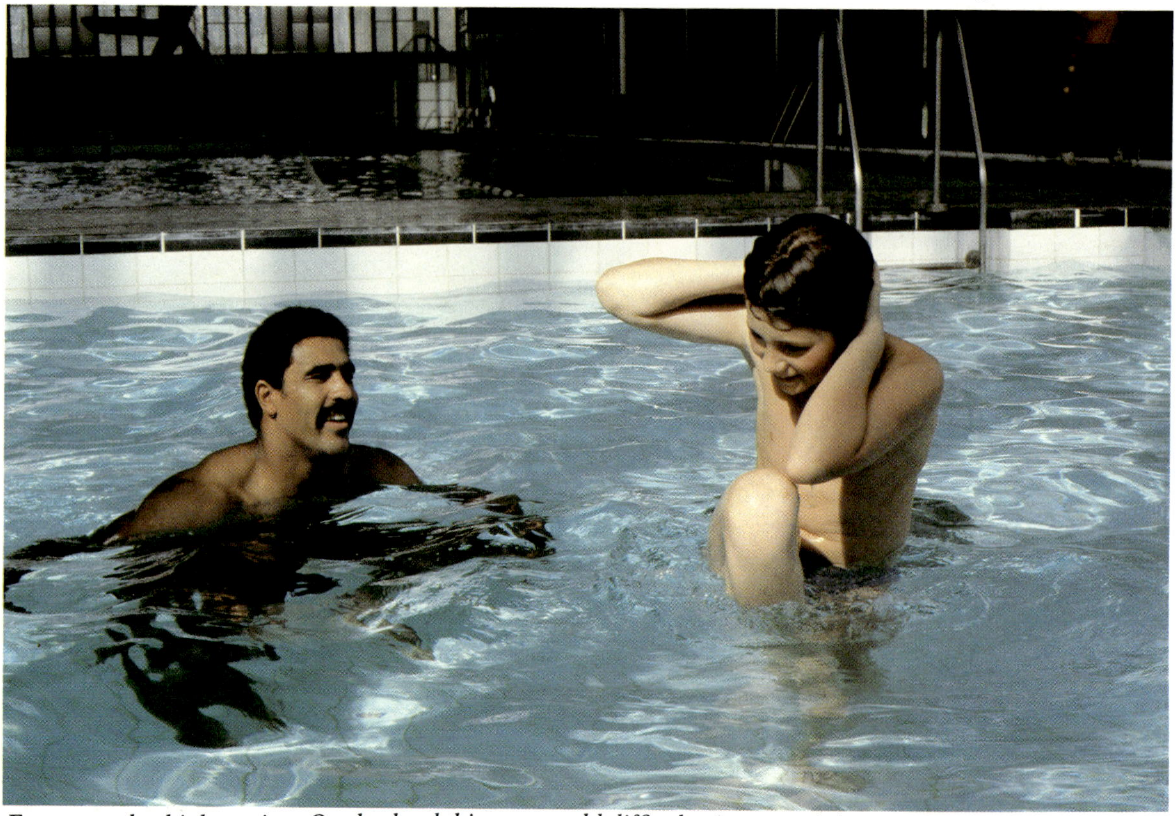

For stomach, thighs, spine. On dry land this one would difficult – in water, it is easy.

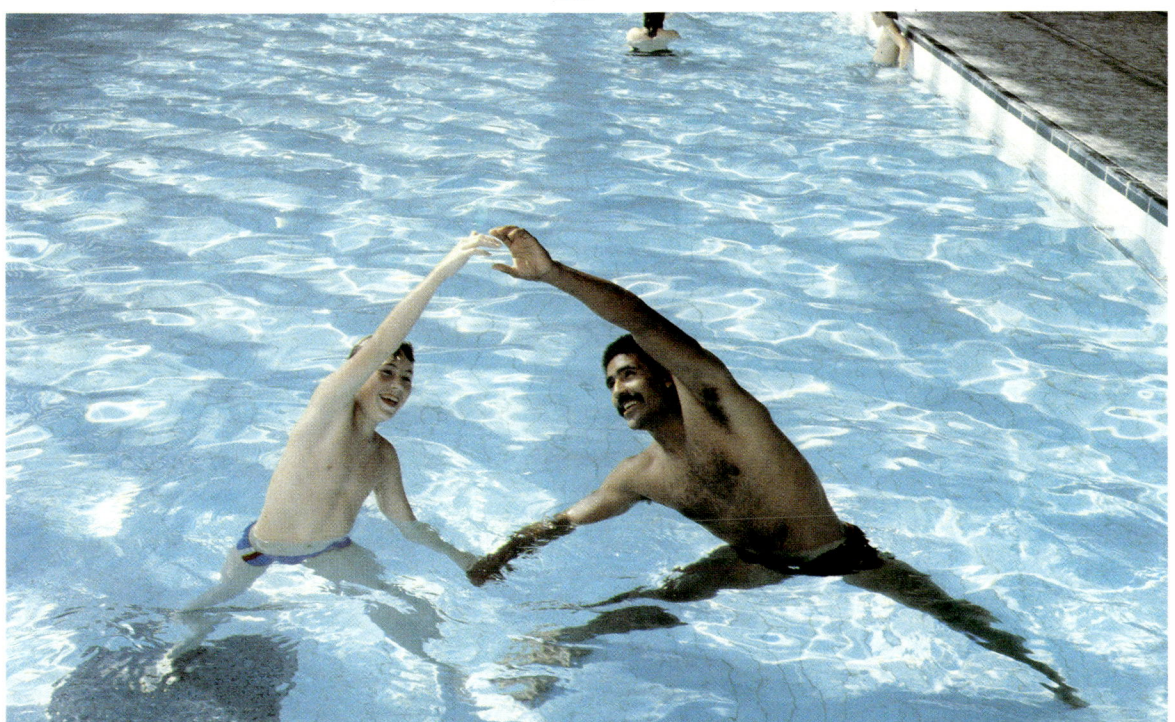

For waistline, ribcage, breathing. Get a partner to join in your water exercises – it does not matter if you are very different heights.

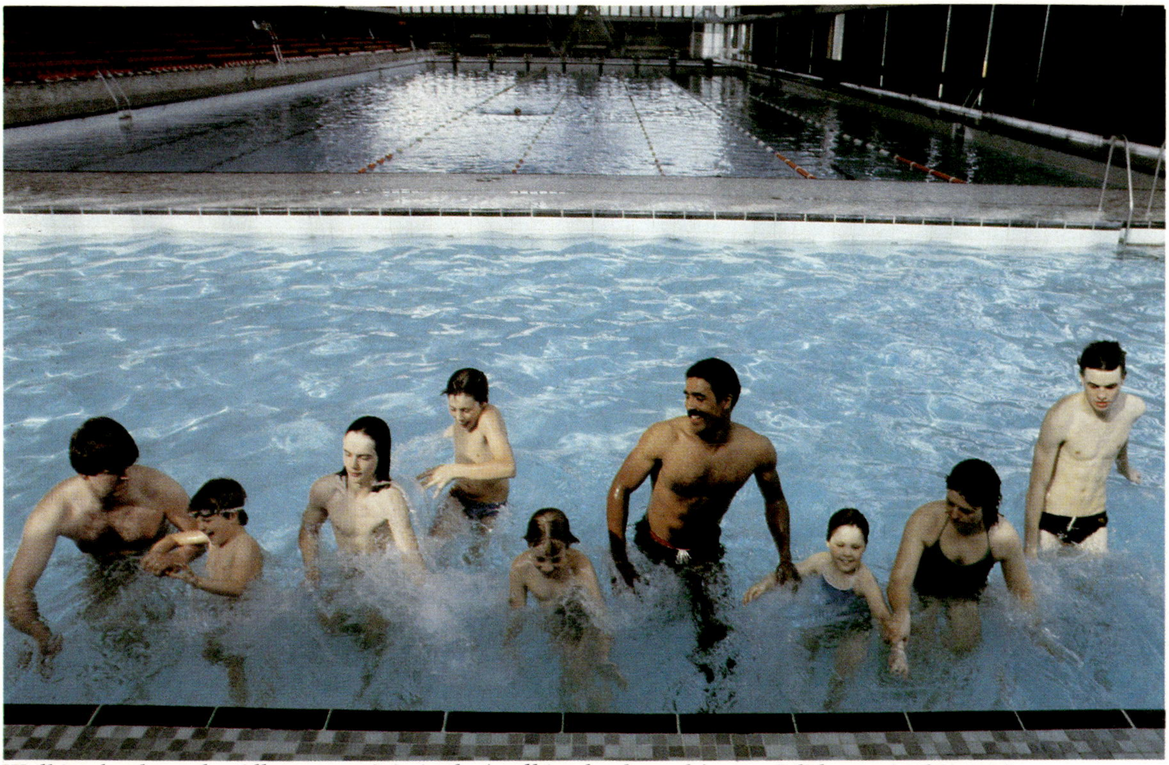

Walking backwards. All ages can join in the 'walking backwards' race. I did not win this one!

BREATHING FOR SWIMMERS

Once you have learnt to swim, a whole new world opens up for you. I was lucky enough to get the chance to go scuba diving in the Cayman Islands last year, and this helped me not just to improve my general swimming ability, but to learn the techniques of correct breathing. During the underwater swimming, I found that because my lungs are so highly developed, I tended to use up more air than most people, which was rather disconcerting for the diving 'buddy' who was meant to share oxygen with me. Anyway, as regards normal swimming, I think that many swimmers could enjoy the activity more if they sorted out their breathing. Here is a guide to correct breathing for the three basic strokes:

Breast-stroke

Breathing is really part of the stroke itself, and is extremely important. You must breathe in when your arms are pulling back, head out of the water, then breathe out during the following leg kick and recovery, as your mouth goes under the water. If you have resisted putting your mouth *under* the water, do practise this – you will not choke, or take in a mouthful, if you remember to breathe *out*, lifting your chin before you breathe in.

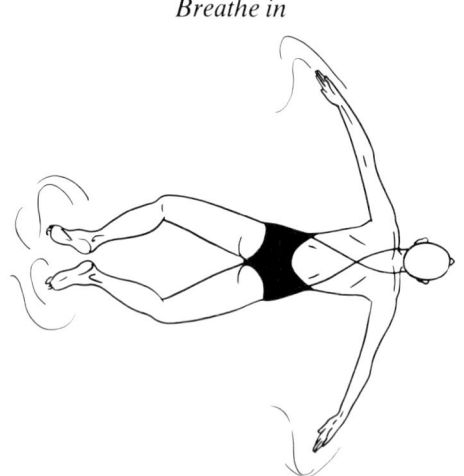

Breathe in

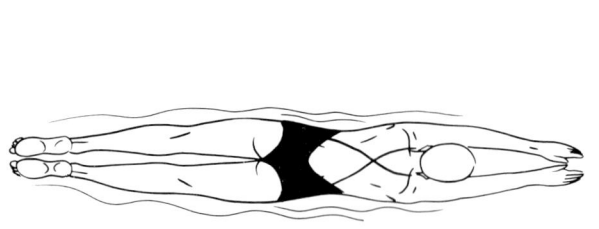

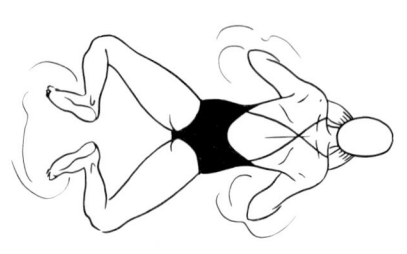

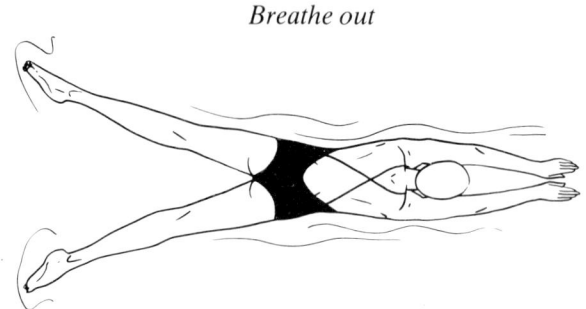

Breathe out

Crawl

Most people find the breathing the most difficult part of this stroke, but if you get it right, it will improve your speed as well as your power. When your left hand enters the water and your right arm is about to come out, you should be in the face down position, mouth closed. As the left arm drives through the stroke, you should blow air *out* through your mouth. Now, your right arm should come forward, starting its downward stroke, while the left elbow breaks the surface. Turn your head to the left and breathe in during the left arm recovery. *Before* the end of the movement, you must complete your breath, and by the time your left hand has entered the water, your face will be down again (mouth closed!). If you find that it is easier for you to turn your head to the right, then you should reverse all these procedures.

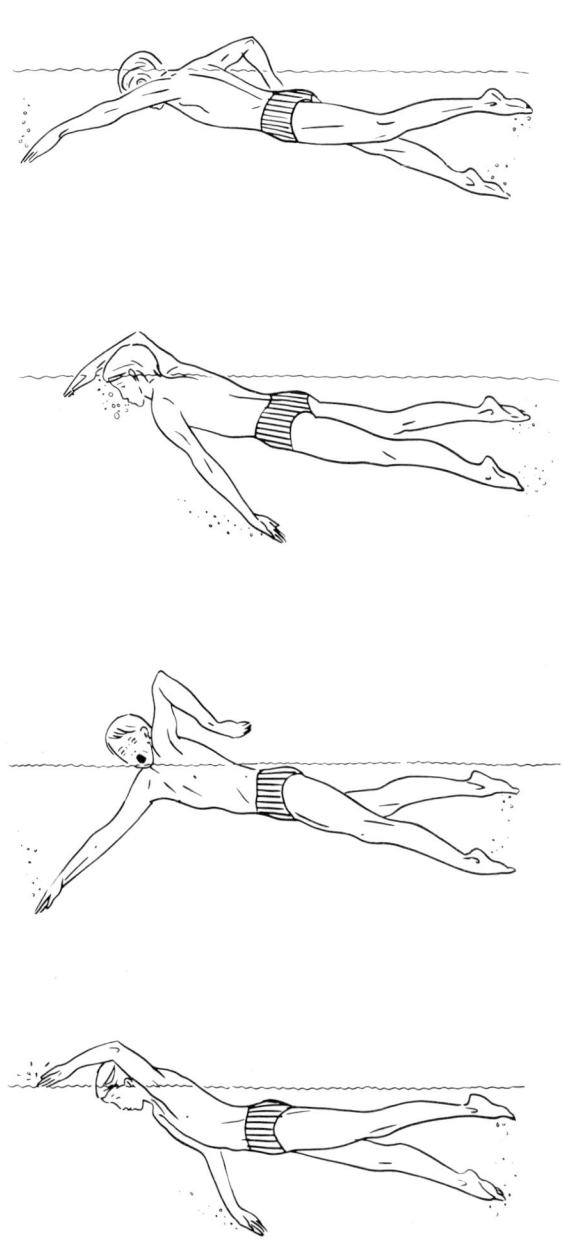

Back-stroke

For the back crawl, try to breathe economically, taking in air, and breathing out through the mouth in a rhythmical movement. If you are doing the English back-stroke, which is really the basis of the life-saving stroke, you must breathe in during the arm recovery, out while the arms are pulling. Remember that all effort, including that exerted in the water, can be aided by breathing *out* during or just before such exertion, *in* during a 'resting' period or glide.

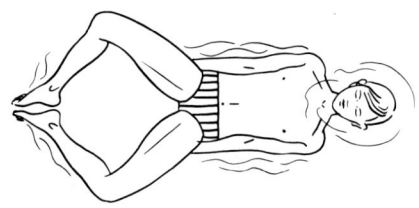

Breathe in

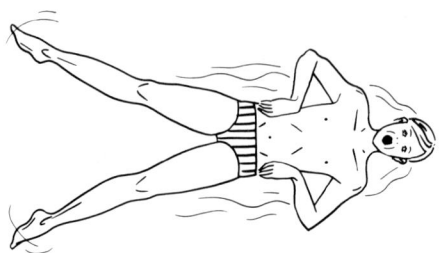

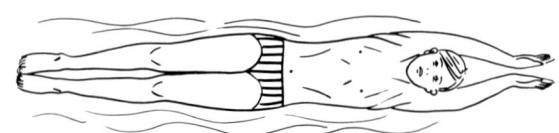

Breathe out

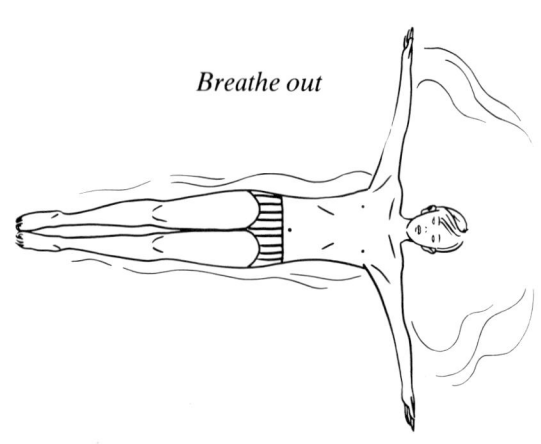

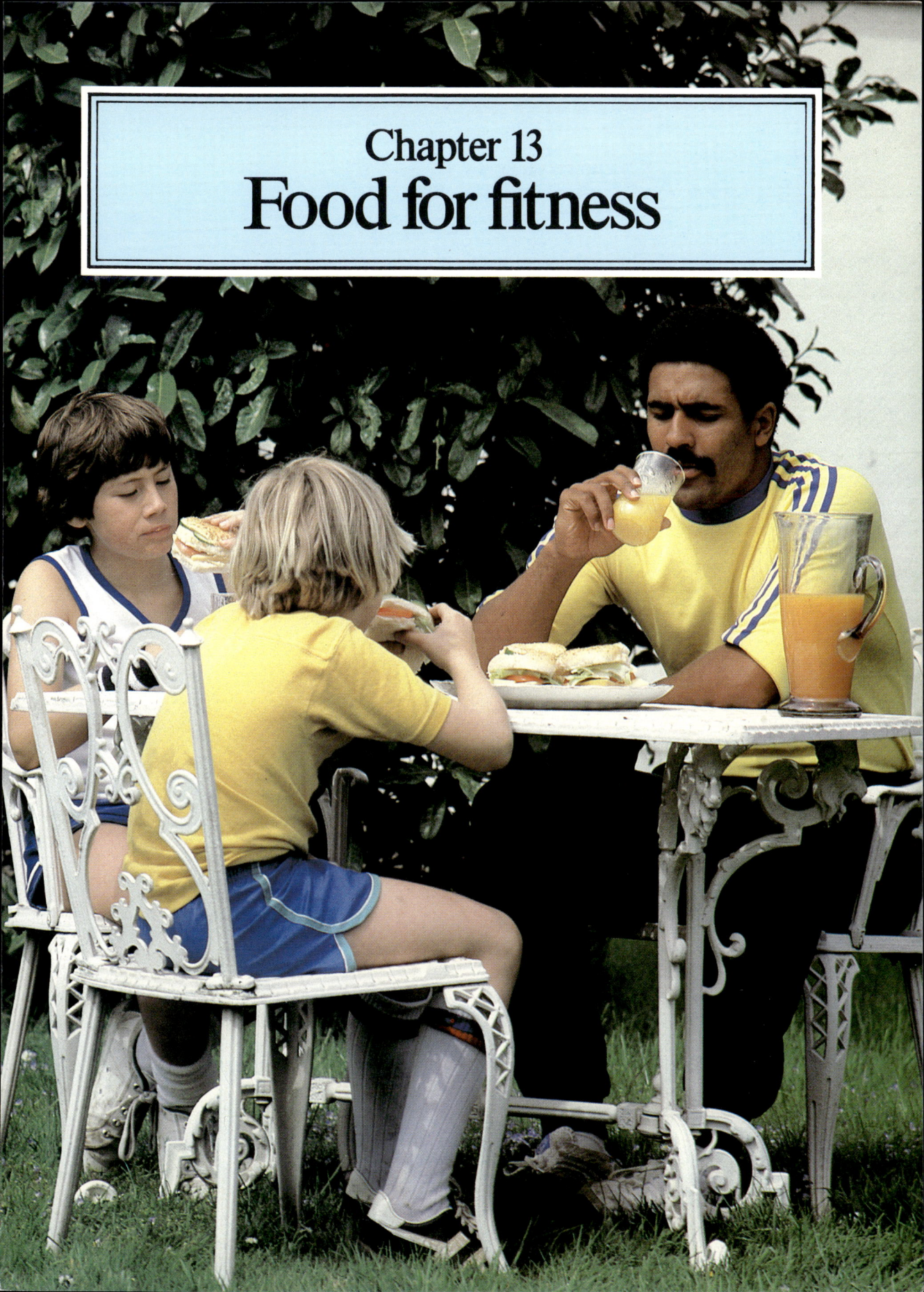

Chapter 13
Food for fitness

People often ask me what kind of diet I follow for decathlon. To be honest, I do not consciously follow any particular diet, although by now I have established an eating pattern which is effective and suits me. I start the day with something simple, not too heavy, to give me energy for training – milk, with cereal, yogurt or both. During the day, I take a break for a cheese roll or sandwich and several soft drinks. Then, after training, I have a bigger meal. I am fond of Big Macs (no chips) if I am out, or a good cooked meat and vegetables meal if I am at home. I eat a lot of fruit, salads, green vegetables and am very keen on raw carrots. I suppose my daily calorie intake must be about 3,000 – which would be excessive for a sedentary worker, but is fine for me. My weight stays at about 13 stones 5 lbs (I am 6' 1" tall) with slight variations. I train all year round, so that any excess calories are quickly burned up as energy.

I do not believe that anyone should ever follow a drastic diet. If you are slightly overweight, just try combining a sensible eating plan with exercise and stand by for dramatic results. It is now known that exercise revs up the calorie burning processes – and this effect continues even *after* the exercise is ended. So, you will lose weight even if you do not alter your diet. If you are very overweight, it makes sense to slim down *before* starting on your exercise programme, otherwise you will put too much strain on your heart, and limbs. (If in doubt, have a check-up.) Never cut right back on carbohydrates (bread, spuds, pasta) when you are exercising. The depletion of liver glycogen in a very low-carbohydrate diet could make it very difficult to generate enough glucose for muscular activity. If you *ever* feel wobbly or faint after your exercise session, do check that diet carefully!

DIETS

Here are four practical diets for people with different nutritional needs. They are meant as a guide only, so if you have any particular health problems or allergies you should check with your doctor before embarking on one of them. They were devised in consultation with Diana MacAdie, an adviser to the Health Education Council.

1 FOR TEENAGE BOYS

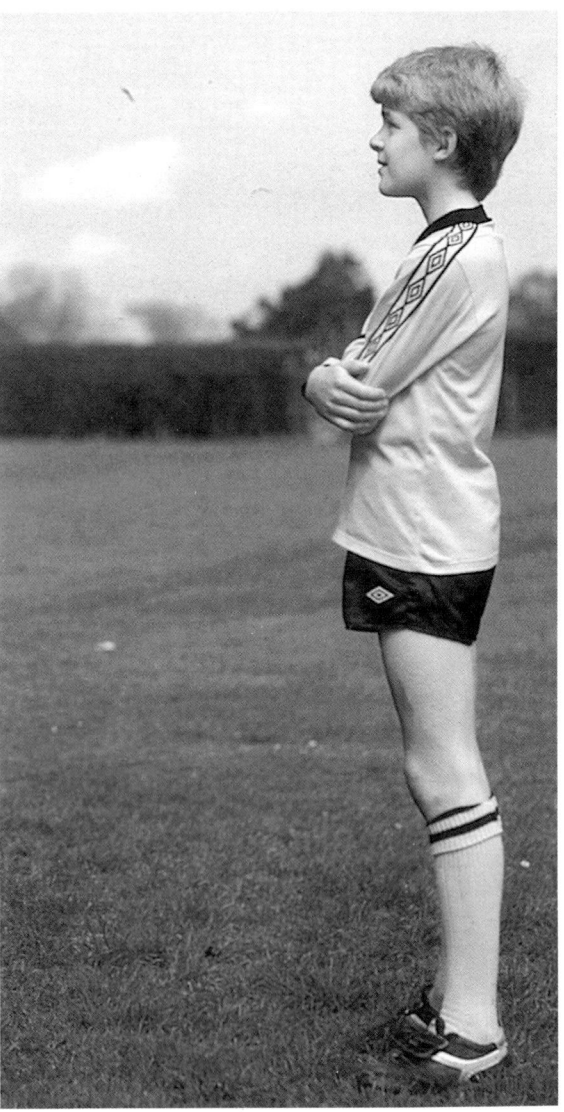

The sports-mad teenage boy needs around 3,000 calories daily to cope with energy output and growth. If he goes to a school where a cafeteria-style lunch is provided, he may miss out on adequate supplies of Vitamin C (in fresh fruit, vegetables), minerals, and even protein, unless steps are taken to ensure that he eats sensibly at breakfast and supper-time. Unfortunately, at lunchtime, he is likely to be faced with a choice of chips, sausages – and more chips! Which is all right – as long as the total menu for the day is balanced out. Useful foods: fresh orange juice, milk, wholemeal bread, wholesome snack-foods like baked beans, eggs, fresh fruit. Danger foods: sugar-loaded soft drinks and sweets which will cause dental decay and leave less room in his stomach for the good foods.

DAILY ALLOWANCES

1 pint whole milk to drink in tea or coffee or as milk-shakes; ½ oz butter or margarine; 4 slices bread, preferably wholemeal.

Breakfast

This is an important meal for the youngster with hard work ahead in the morning and only a little protein food until suppertime. It does not have to be cooked – choose one of the following:

a Bowl of muesli or other cereal topped with chopped banana, milk from allowance and very little sugar; slice of wholemeal toast with Marmite; fruit yoghurt; tea or coffee.

b 2 eggs, scrambled with sweetcorn, served on 1 slice wholemeal toast, topped with sliced tomatoes; fresh unsweetened orange juice; extra slice toast with honey; tea or coffee.

c Hi-energy milk-shake: whisk together orange-flavoured fruit yoghurt, 1 cup milk, 1 egg, 2 tbs orange juice, and serve frothy with a little nutmeg on top and a couple of wholemeal biscuits for dunking.

d Bacon sandwich: grill two slices lean bacon, and serve in a sandwich of wholemeal bread with sliced tomato; fresh unsweetened pineapple or orange juice; 1 apple; tea or coffee.

e Egg dip: whisk two small eggs and soak 1 slice wholemeal bread in the mixture, turning once. Fry lightly in vegetable oil. Serve with sweetcorn, grilled tomatoes. 1 orange in segments; tea or coffee.

Although lots of youngsters resist breakfast, none of these meals takes long to prepare – and the results are worth it. Set the table the night before, set the alarm fifteen minutes earlier, and serve the food attractively. Encourage older children to do their own cooking if possible.

Lunch

If he eats school meals, then he should know what to choose. Avoid too much stodge, chips or confectionery.

Packed lunch ideas

If he takes a packed lunch to school, here are some packed lunch ideas:

Use two slices wholemeal bread for sandwiches and try these fillings: mashed sardines, lemon juice and tomatoes; peanut butter; cheese and Marmite with cress; scrambled eggs mixed with sweetcorn and a little tomato ketchup. You could also add cooked chicken drumstick with 'dip' of pickle or relish; fruit yoghurt; grapes; apples; satsumas (easier to peel than oranges); wedges of cheese for nibbling; frozen cans of fruit juice (thawed and still cold by lunchtime); Kit-Kat or other chocolate bar. Avoid too many crisps which are salt- and fat-loaded, put children off eating other foods, and are not a good snack choice. Cheesy biscuits or wholemeal crackers are better.

After school

If he is off to training or to practice in the evening, it can be a real boost if he has an easily-digested snack immediately after school: a bowl of cereal with fruit and honey, a Mars bar, or honey sandwich, washed down with fruit juice or water will help push up energy levels until suppertime.

Supper

This is the meal when everyone should take stock of what has been eaten during the rest of the day – and fill the gaps. Here are some ideas:

LIGHT SUPPERS

(for youngsters who have already eaten a proper three-course school lunch or substantial packed lunch)

a 2 frozen beefburgers, small portion baked beans, or peas; fruit salad.

b Cheesy baked potato: 1 large jacket spud, centre scooped out mixed with grated Cheddar, re-heated, and served with salad; 1 apple.

c 4 fish fingers, grilled tomatoes, sweetcorn; apple pureé with yoghurt.

d Open sandwich: 1 slice wholemeal bread topped with lettuce, cottage cheese or cream cheese, peach halves, cucumber, watercress; milk-shake.

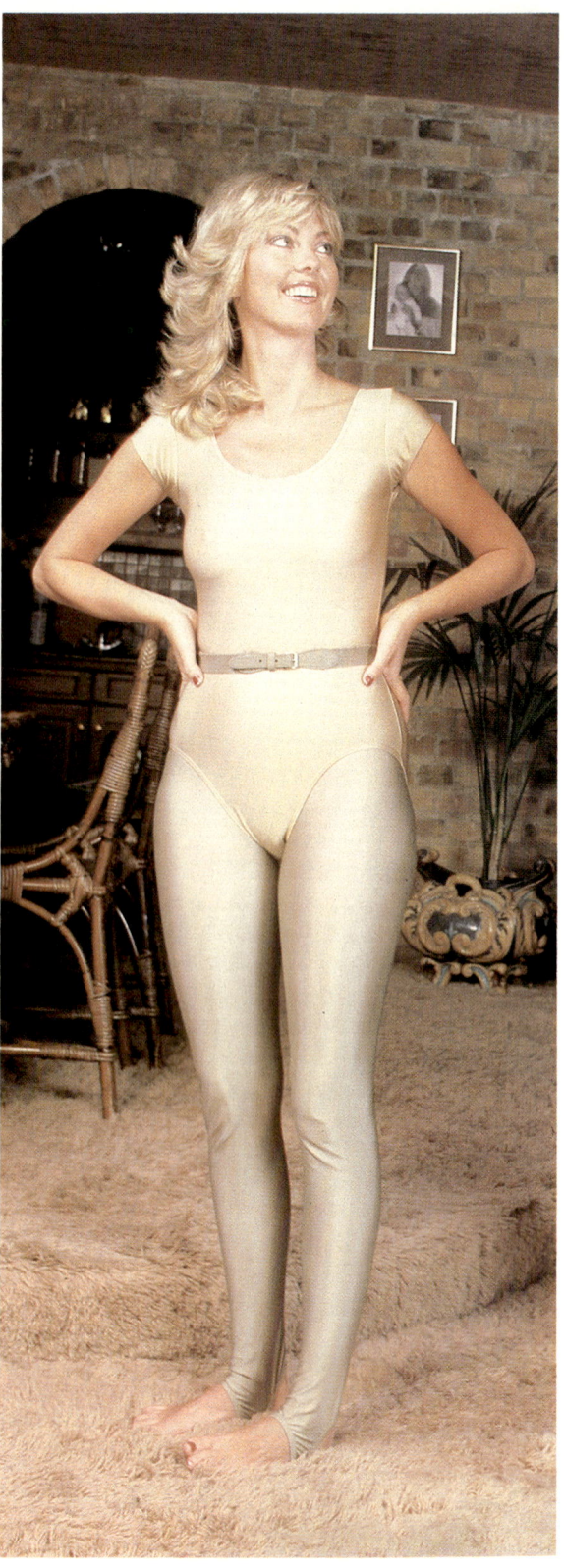
SUBSTANTIAL SUPPERS

(for youngsters who have had a snack lunch only)

a Shepherd's pie with grated cheese on top; cabbage, carrots, green beans; wholemeal apple pie, custard.

b Cod or coley cooked in mushroom soup with onion, sweetcorn, boiled new potatoes with skins on, or chips, peas; chopped banana with ice-cream and chocolate sauce.

c Chinese dinner: stir-fry chicken breast or leg in very little oil, then add finely chopped onion, mushrooms, carrots, beansprouts, and toss until cooked but not mushy – stir in a little soy sauce and serve with rice; fresh fruit salad with lychees (canned) and ice-cream.

d Casseroled leg of beef with carrots, onions, mashed potatoes, cabbage or broccoli; fruit yoghurt with an extra handful of raisins and nuts stirred in (serve in a bowl for a change).

Pre-match meals

If Saturday is his big sports day, plan the day's meals so that the menu a couple of hours before the game is high-carbohydrate, *not* high-protein. He needs: cereal with fruit and milk, a honey sandwich, or chip butty with an apple. Have the main, cooked dinner after the game. Drink fruit juice and water in the morning, a soft drink before the game – milk *afterwards*.

2 FOR TEENAGE GIRLS AND WOMEN WITHOUT A WEIGHT PROBLEM

Teenage girls need about 2,100 calories daily – the same as a woman who is active (even if she is in a sedentary job, and she takes exercise regularly) and has no weight problem. The girl's needs are just a little different – she should have additional milk or cheese products for calcium to ensure healthy bones and teeth, and protein (in fish, meat, eggs) for growth. Iron is a very important nutritional requirement – during menstruation, iron is lost, so that all young women do need to make sure they include plenty of iron-containing food in their diet. Anorexia Nervosa is prevalent among young girls who become obsessed with dieting. It is important to emphasise the benefits to young girls of good nutrition. Exercise will help you keep in shape, and there really is no need to go on a faddish diet during your teens. But it is also daft to subsist on a diet of junk food and sweets. They will make you look awful, and feel it too. Useful foods: liver, eggs, green vegetables, meat (all good sources of iron), wholesome sandwiches, water and mineral water, wholegrain cereals, fruit, cheese. Danger foods: sweets, greasy foods like chips and fry-ups (bad for complexion).

DAILY ALLOWANCES

1 pint whole milk for teenage girls, ½ pint for women (for use in tea or coffee); ½ oz butter or margarine; 2 slices bread, preferably wholemeal.

Breakfast

Even if you are in a rush, you should not miss out on breakfast. Choose one of the following quick-to-serve ideas:

a Unsweetened fruit juice; poached egg on 1 slice wholemeal toast; natural yoghurt.
b Whisk together small carton natural yoghurt with juice of 1 fresh orange and 1 egg; toast and butter from allowance.
c Grapefruit juice; grilled kidneys on 1 slice toast from allowance; grilled tomatoes.
d Small portion unsweetened muesli with chopped apple and nuts on top, milk from allowance; slice toast from allowance with Marmite or Bovril.
e Unsweetened orange juice; 2 eggs, scrambled, with bread and butter from allowance.

Lunch

Take a packed lunch to school or work if you can. Here are some ideas:

a 2 slices lean ham; large mixed salad; slice of bread and butter; 1 orange or banana.
b Tuna fish sandwich with bread from allowance, lemon juice and watercress; grapes or pear.
c Hard-boiled egg; mixed salad of watercress, tomatoes, grated carrot, nuts, lemon juice dressing; bread and butter from allowance.
d Small carton cottage cheese on bed of lettuce topped with sliced grapefruit and orange; bread and butter from allowance, spread with Marmite.

e Open sandwich: lettuce with cubes of cheese, celery, chopped apple in a dressing of diet mayonnaise on 1 slice wholemeal bread; small carton fruit yoghurt.

If you have to eat in a canteen or restaurant go for salads, egg dishes, or meat dishes with a side salad instead of chips.

Supper

Make up any nutritional deficiencies of the day with a well thought-out supper. Choose one portion of liver or red meat every other day.

a Small grilled mackerel, french beans, salad; bread and butter from allowance; small piece of cheese.
b Grilled liver with tomatoes, orange slices and sauce, large portion green vegetables, 1 small potato; creme caramel.
c Chicken leg marinated in lemon juice, grilled and served with spinach and tomatoes, jacket potato; fruit yoghurt.
d Well-grilled lean lamb chop or small steak with jacket potato, mixed salad; fresh fruit and ice-cream.
e 2 slices roast meat (lean), cabbage, carrots, cauliflower; apple crumble.

Pre-sport snacks

Cereal, with milk and fruit, fresh fruit with yoghurt, or a health-food store cereal 'bar', will help bridge the gap between work or school and evening sport. But do not eat *too* near the time of your match or practice – women, unfortunately, have a longer 'digestion period' than men simply because they are usually smaller. (If you are a large lady, ignore this advice!) After a match, do make up energy and iron stores with a good meal (even if you cannot face it until the next day, make sure that your very next main meal is a suitably well-balanced one).

3 FOR TRIM, ATHLETIC MEN – OR THOSE WHO WANT TO BE TRIM AND ATHLETIC

Most men need between 2,500 and 3,000 calories a day, depending on their job and the amount of exercise they take. A lot has been written about

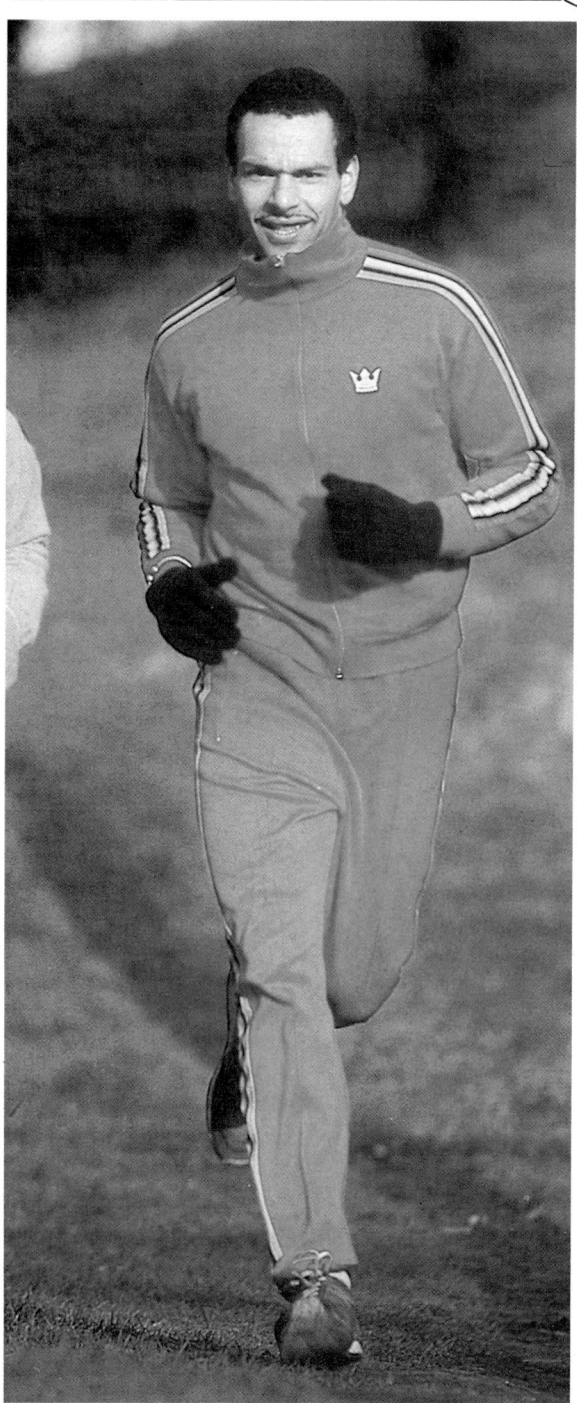

foods, and try to keep alcohol down to a sensible level – ½ bottle of wine or 2 pints of beer a day is fine, more is excessive. Useful foods: fish, cooked simply, with no fancy sauces, lean meats, jacket potatoes (no butter), wholemeal sandwiches, fruit. Danger foods: pub snacks like bangers, curries, and shepherd's pie, take-aways, alcohol.

DAILY ALLOWANCES

½ pint milk or 1 pint low-fat milk for tea or coffee; ½ oz butter or margarine (polyunsaturated if you like). Beware of fry-ups, which are fat-loaded. Buy high-fibre cereals.

Breakfast

a Fresh unsweetened orange juice; wholemeal bread with cottage cheese and tomato.
b Stewed fruit; grilled kidney or lean bacon; slice of toast from allowance; grilled tomatoes.
c Orange and grapefruit segments; grilled mushrooms on toast from allowance with poached egg; sweetcorn.
d Muesli with grated apple and yoghurt on top; sprinkling of All-bran.
e ½ grapefruit; poached haddock with tomato; bread and butter from allowance.

Lunch

Choose a packed lunch which includes fresh fruit, sandwiches using fish, tinned fish or lean meat, salad. Or, go for one of these restaurant ideas:
a Slice of melon; 1 slice lean roast beef with mixed salad; bread and butter from allowance.
b Clear soup; grilled white fish with tomatoes, green salad; small portion ice-cream.
c Grilled liver and lean bacon, green vegetables, boiled potatoes; fresh fruit salad.

Supper

If you have a big meal at lunchtime, you do *not* need another one in the evening. Do not let the lady in your life kill you with good intentions – you do not need jam roly-poly or stew with dumplings. Choose a simple, tasty meal and if you are eating out go for the light foods, not the heavy over-seasoned ones.
a Cucumber, melon and chopped tomato salad tossed in lemon juice, tarragon vinegar and chopped

low-cholesterol diets – unless your doctor has put you on a specific diet, it is a good idea to follow one which is low in all forms of fat, high in dietary fibre, and which contains a variety of foods. Resist overcooked, over-sauced, over-seasoned restaurant

mint; lean lamb chop, broccoli, new potatoes.
b Small avocado with lemon juice; grilled herring or mackerel, green salad; orange mousse.
c Raw mushroom salad with soy sauce and spring onion dressing; cauliflower cheese, grilled tomatoes, jacket potato.
d Half grapefruit; grilled chicken with tarragon and brown rice; tomato salad.
e Lean beef stew, carrots, tomatoes, parsley; baked apple with raisins and nuts.

Pre-sport snacks

Small sandwich or roll (must be at least two hours beforehand), or fresh fruit with bread and butter from allowance, or cereal with fruit and nuts. After sport beware of boozing too much. For every pint of lager, drink one of water. Drink water *before* the first lager, to quench your thirst, otherwise you will not actually *taste* the first alcoholic drink and will immediately crave another one.

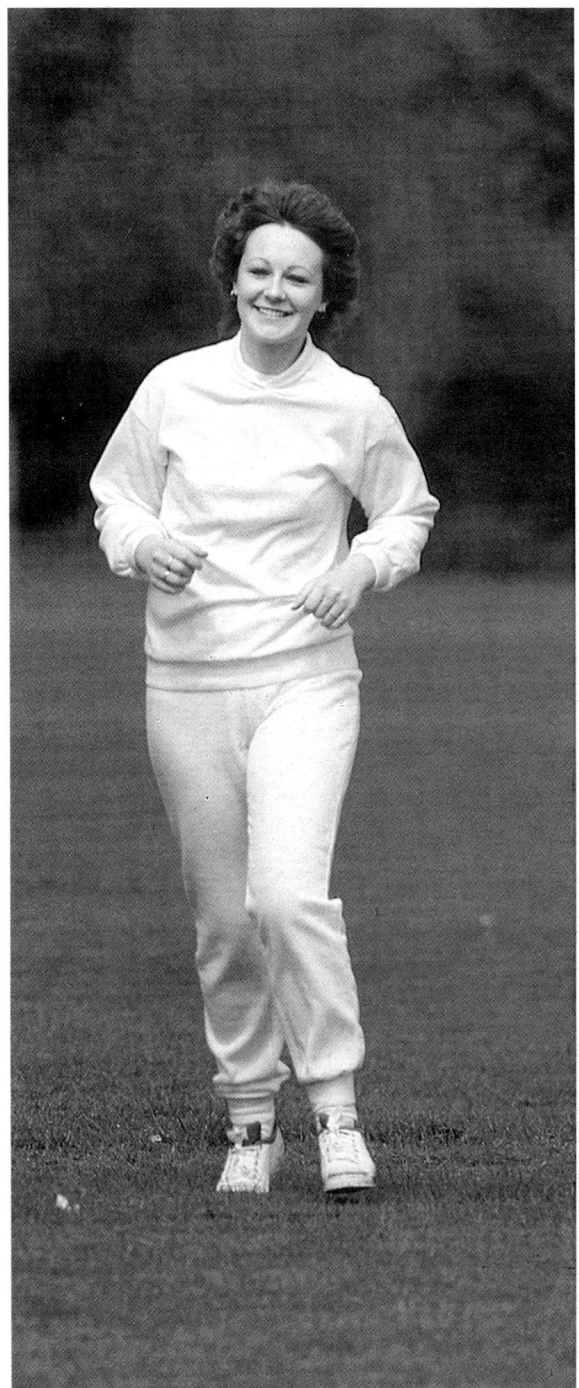

4 FOR WEIGHT-CONSCIOUS WOMEN

Never go below 1,500 calories daily if you are combining your slimming campaign with a sporty one. You really do need to make sure your diet is rich in iron, fresh vegetables and fruit, protein – and adequate carbohydrate too. Keep your energy up by eating small, regular meals instead of a few big ones. Useful foods: fruit, open sandwiches, slimmer's foods like low-calorie soups and salad dressings, natural yoghurt, wholemeal bread which actually fills you up much better than slimmer's bread for very few additional calories. Danger foods: sweets, greasy foods, diet 'aids' like slimming biscuits, drinks and puddings. Try this six-meal a day plan, making sure that exercise is taken at least two hours after a meal.

Choose six meals from this list:
★ Poached egg on wholemeal toast, 1 orange.
★ Small portion grilled liver, green salad.
★ Slimmer's soup, wholemeal bread and butter or low-fat spread, natural yoghurt.
★ Small tin baked beans on 1 slice wholemeal toast with sliced tomatoes.
★ Lean lamb chop, large portion green vegetables, 1 orange.
★ 1 apple, cottage cheese on wholemeal bread with cucumber and lettuce, plus low-calorie dressing.
★ 2 slices lean roast turkey or chicken, thin gravy, small boiled potato, grilled tomatoes.

★ Large portion fresh fruit salad with natural yoghurt and wheat germ on top.

★ Small portion bran cereal with banana and a little skimmed milk, 1 slice wholemeal bread and low-fat spread.

★ 2 fish fingers, well grilled, large mixed salad with low-calorie dressing.

★ 2-egg omelette with herbs, spinach or broccoli, 1 pear.

★ Small, lean steak, jacket potato, salad.

★ Any grilled or steamed white fish with mushrooms, braised celery or coleslaw (low-calorie dressing), grilled tomatoes.

Drinks

Allow ½ pint milk, or 1 pint low-fat milk daily, and drink lots of water and mineral water to refresh you after exercising. If you feel a bit droopy, do take a multi-vitamin pill containing iron daily.

Once you have achieved the weight you desire, go on to diet 2 or a similar, sensible, diet-plan.

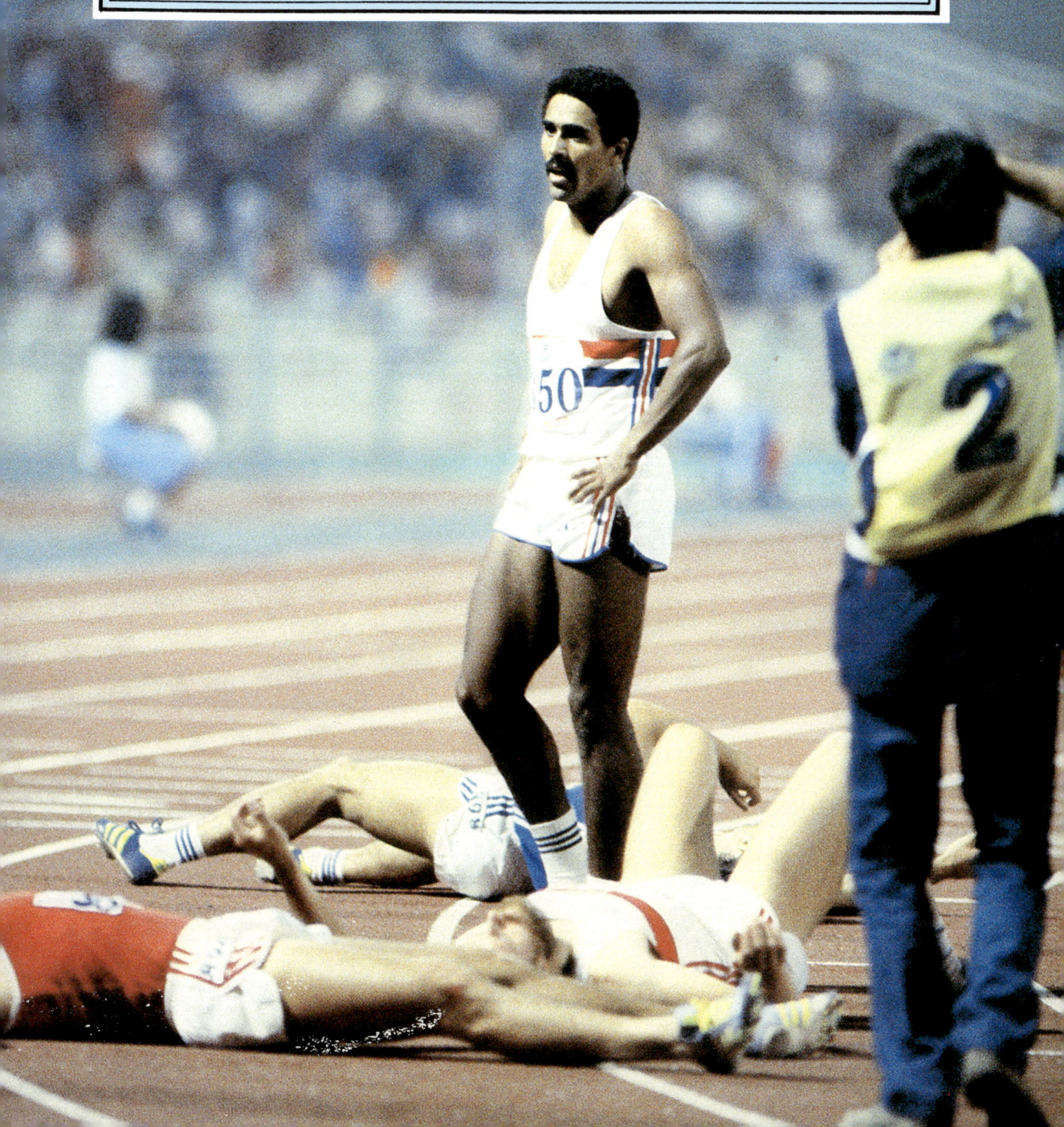

Chapter 14
Planning a fitness campaign

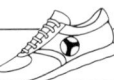

When I enter a big competition, I immediately start to plan my fitness campaign with meticulous attention to detail. It is a scientifically worked-out programme devised in consultation with my coach and the specialists who advise me on the various events.

The plan consists of a thirty-five week chart, culminating in the competition itself. The four main areas of work are *strength, speed, endurance,* and *skill* – the same four for all ten events in the decathlon. I work out my plan backwards from the competition, allowing three to four days at the very end for recovery and restful preparation. I spend the first ten weeks of the campaign on strength (with exercises like bounding in a weighted jacket – see page 92), and endurance (sit-ups, press-ups, pull-ups to increase my staying-power, plus sprints in groups with a brief rest between each group). After about six weeks, I start on the technical work – perfecting the technique on shot putt, discus, pole vault, high jump, and the short run-ups which are so important in some of the events. About eight to ten weeks before the competition it is all systems go with speed training – sprint starts – making sure I am as fast as possible! For the last five or six weeks, I try to do everything as perfectly as possible before that thirty-five week deadline.

I keep a highly detailed diary of daily, weekly, and monthly progress, and charts showing what I have still to achieve. No one understands them apart from me and I am sure that if I fed them into a computer it would explode. When you are dealing with details like timing (a few tenths of a second can make all the difference to your performance in the track events), your diary and charts assume an almost religious importance. I am also very wary about divulging all the secrets of my training programme – there are spies everywhere! Seriously, I think non-athletes would probably be very surprised at just how much mathematical skill goes into preparing my training schedules. I am convinced that many sports enthusiasts could do much better in their chosen sport if they actually sat down and planned ahead more carefully, bearing in mind their own strengths and weaknesses.

As a great planner myself, I suggest that *you* follow suit, whether you want to get into shape for a match, an important event (a wedding, perhaps?), or just a holiday when you want to look and feel your best. Here are some ideas:

YOUR AIM

First of all decide what you are aiming to achieve. Do you want to clip a few seconds, or even minutes off a specific running time? Do you aim just to finish a marathon or fun run in a fairly decent time? Do you want to play brilliantly in the final of your school house soccer match, with a vast improvement in all your skills? Do you want to sock-it-to-'em in the knock-out darts competition at the pub? Do you aim to lose two stones before your holiday in July, *and* get rid of your stomach bulge? Do you want to feel fighting fit before you start the new term at university? Whatever it is – *write it down!* Make sure that your aim is definitely within the realms of possibility – there is nothing more depressing than aiming *so* high that you are doomed to be disappointed, however hard you train. When I am planning my own fitness campaign, I am always realistic. Remember that you can always improve that little bit more during your next concentrated effort. This time, though, make it *possible.*

AREAS OF WORK

Now think about the specific areas you need to concentrate on during your pre-event training. For athletes, soccer players, runners, ball-players, the areas are likely to be very much the same as mine: strength, speed, endurance, and skill. There may perhaps be some additional specific aspects which you need to polish up – for instance, your psychological attitude, or confidence. Do not forget that confidence only comes when you know you are doing well (if you are confident and you are *not* physically able to cope, then you have a problem! In the early days of the marathon popularity explosion, there were some entrants who had a kind of mad confidence based on hope, lack of knowledge, and sheer bravado. They usually came unstuck. Luckily, that kind of daft attitude is now largely disappearing as the word gets around that marathon running is extremely hard work.) Or, there may be some specific area or skill which you really need to improve – heading techniques for soccer players, accuracy for ping-pong fiends, the way your bottom wobbles in a bikini for holiday fitness freaks. Decide what these areas of work are – and, again – *write them down!*

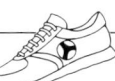

THE TIME AVAILABLE

Now consult your diary for the all-important ingredient in your fitness campaign – the time at your disposal. This is obviously going to be a very important factor in your plan, and affect the way you organise your life. If your time is short, and you have a lot to do, then try to allot as much space as possible in your daily schedule for your fitness campaign. Let the dust gather, the car get dirty, the grass grow high in the garden, if your time for fitness is short – or make your domestic problems fit in with your campaign by becoming part of it: do exercises while you do your housework, stretching routines while you wash the car, endurance tests while pushing the mower.

PLAN OUT THE CAMPAIGN

Start by working backwards from the 'event', allowing a day or so for 'R and R'. I do *not* believe in working flat out until the big day – you will just become tired, fed-up and thoroughly bored by the whole thing. I believe that the body needs a little break to adjust before the event, and the brain definitely works better on the big day if it is left alone to do some bright computing with no more information being fed in for about twenty-four hours beforehand. Exams experts always advise candidates to study hard up until twenty-four hours or so before the exam, then take a breather while the brain sorts out all the information. Bearing in mind that the brain is also responsible for your *bodily* co-ordination, your muscle power, your determination, it makes sense to cash in on any unseen work which your very own built-in motivating machine is able to do for you!

Concentrate the most time on your weaknesses, but also allow adequate time to polish up your strong points. Remember that it takes much longer to build up muscular strength and endurance than other things – that is why I spend longer on these areas. It is no good realising a week before a ten-mile fun run that your running style is wonderful, but you really need to be able to last out for longer than the five miles that you are currently able to run!

Here are six sample charts to give you an idea of how to plan your own campaign:

1 *30-year-old club runner, male*

AIM: To run in 20 km (12 mile) cross-country club event.

AREAS OF WORK: Strength and endurance need building up – previous experience only 15 km (9 miles). General fitness level good, plays squash twice weekly, drinks very little, good diet.

TIME AVAILABLE: 2 months to the event. Has 1 hour available after work on weekday evenings, Saturday and Sunday afternoons.

PLAN OF CAMPAIGN: Bounding and leg strengthening exercises (p. 92, 94) during the week, plus squash for variety. Building up endurance with fairly long runs on Saturday and Sunday afternoons, varying terrain. After one month, introduce *Fartlek* (p. 66) on Saturday afternoons, and shorter runs with a rest between them in the evenings at a local track. More distance work during fifth and sixth weeks, and aim to hit that top distance around seventh week, with a much lighter work-load on the eighth week.

2 *15-year-old school football player, male*

AIM: To play well in important school fixture – position, midfield.

AREAS OF WORK: Basic four, plus special attention needed on ball control, heading, marking. Has weekly half-day school football, and gym.

TIME AVAILABLE: 2 weeks to the event. 2 hours daily available after school and before homework, plus Sunday afternoons (works Saturday).

PLAN OF CAMPAIGN: Start with ball control, heading, marking practice (p. 98) after school, and use gym lessons for leg-strengthening and agility exercises (pp. 92, 94). Play a game on Sunday afternoon, concentrating on tactics, position, skills, team-work. Watch diet closely (p. 116) during the two-week pre-match build-up.

3 *12-year-old school swimmer, female*

AIM: To swim 1 mile for charity in pool.

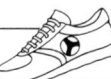

AREAS OF WORK: Strength, endurance, breathing, style (especially for *economy* as the swimmer in question tends to splash about a lot). Her diet is one area which could be improved, too – tends to be high on carbs, fats, low on protein foods.

TIME AVAILABLE: 3 weeks to the event. 1 hour training in school pool twice a week, 1 hour after school at home or in the garden if it is fine, 2 hours in the pool on Sundays.

PLAN OF CAMPAIGN: Use school training time to brush up on style and breathing (pp. 112–114), then practise these on Sundays alone in the pool. Use skipping exercises (p. 25), and do leg and arm strengthening routines (pp. 45, 71–82, 92) at home after school. Make a real effort to eat more protein, fresh fruits, vegetables, less junk food (p. 118).

4 45-year-old tennis player, male

AIM: To play in mixed doubles match to start club knock-out competition – was knocked out in first round last year.

AREAS OF WORK: Basic four, plus service (a lot of improvement necessary – this was weak point last year), volleying close to the net, accurate smashing, backhand. Might help a lot if rich lunches were cut down a bit, too!

TIME AVAILABLE: 6 weeks to the match, 2 hours training with partner on court on Saturday afternoons, 1 hour after work in the evening (no partner, but a good wall available).

PLAN OF CAMPAIGN: Try cycling or jogging to the court every day. Use Saturday afternoon sessions on court to brush up that service, volleying and backhand with partner, and supplement this with evening practice alone. Use lunch hours for some weights exercises (pp. 71–82) (easy to bring dumb-bells to work), cutting down on actual eating time.

5 30-year-old unfit sedentary worker, female

AIM: To lose 9.53 kg (1½ stones) in time for summer holiday in Miami and become fit enough to enjoy swimming, sailing, tennis.

AREAS OF WORK: General, plus special problem with fat stomach, thighs (through sitting down so much). Also very rarely walks, and needs to get in

some swimming practice and build up strength for sailing and tennis. Junk food diet needs sorting out!

TIME AVAILABLE: 2 months to the holiday. Could spare 2 hours once a week for swimming, Saturday and Sunday mornings for general exercising. Apart from that – no time!

PLAN OF CAMPAIGN: Start on good 1,500 calories daily diet (p. 121), progressing up to 1,800 calories daily diet as exercise is increased. During the weekly swim, include a few pool exercises (pp. 108–111). Try a gentle jog on Saturdays, strengthening and firming exercises on Sunday mornings (pp. 71–82), and isometrics (p. 48) to tone up muscles at work. In the second month, increase running distance, exercise repeats, and concentrate on stomach and thigh muscle exercises (pp. 37, 41–45, 86, 88).

6 25-year-old unfit sales representative, male

AIM: To get in shape for wedding and honeymoon in Greece – fianceé is keen windsurfer who plans to introduce him to this sport. Does not want to look a fool! Would like to lose 6.35 kg (1 stone), shape up and get fit fast!

AREAS OF WORK: Flabby stomach needs flattening, legs and arms need strengthening for windsurfing, plus back, co-ordination, balance. Diet needs stringent action – now largely consists of pub lunches and take-aways.

TIME AVAILABLE: 2 months to holiday. Weekday evenings only available as he has working weekends. Could spare 2 hours twice a week, plus half-hour workout nightly at home, perhaps a short jog in the morning.

PLAN OF CAMPAIGN: Enrol in gym near work, and spend 2 hours twice weekly on weights and general exercise. Pub lunches to be replaced by gentle jog in the park, followed by wholesome nibble and mineral water at desk. In the evenings, the twenty-minute workout 2 (p. 41) could gradually give way in the second month to exercises concentrating more on mobility, skill and co-ordination (pp. 104, 106), and football exercises to help leg and feet control (pp. 92–98). An intake of around 1,500 calories daily for the 2 months will yield substantial weight loss (p. 121).

Reference

Write to the addresses below for more information on sport and fitness. Although many of the addresses are in London, they can put you in touch with local contacts. Sports shops are also a good starting point for information, especially the large Olympus chain with over sixty branches. The YMCA and Central Council of Physical Recreation are also very helpful, and the latter can give information on *all* forms of sport and exercise, including dance.

SPORTS GOVERNING BODIES

The Sports Council,
16 Upper Woburn Place,
London WC1

Scottish Sports Council,
1 St Colme Street,
Edinburgh,
Scotland

Athletics

Amateur Athletic Association
(England & Wales),
Francis House,
Francis Street,
London SW1

British Marathon Runners
Club,
22 Mount Avenue,
Stone,
Staffs

British Sports Association for
the Disabled,
Stoke Mandeville Stadium,
Harvey Road,
Aylesbury,
Bucks

Central Council of Physical
Recreation,
Francis House,
Francis Street,
London SW1

Cycling

British Cycling Federation,
16 Upper Woburn Place,
London WC1

Dance & movement

Keep Fit Association,
16 Upper Woburn Place,
London WC1

Women's League of Health &
Beauty,
1 The Ridge,
Newton Solney,
Nr Burton-on-Trent,
Staffs

Football

The Football Association,
16 Lancaster Gate,
London W2

Women's Football
Association,
11 Portsea Mews,
Portsea Place,
London W2

Golf

English Golf Union,
12a Denmark Street,
Wokingham,
Berks

Jogging

National Jogging Association,
35 Bruton Street,
London W1

National Jogging Club,
114 Bond Street,
London W1

Lawn Tennis

All England Lawn Tennis &
Croquet Club,
Church Road,
Wimbledon,
London SW1

Veterans' Lawn Tennis
Association of GB,
Olde Forge Cottage,
140 Braywick Road,
Maidenhead,
Berks

Squash

Squash Rackets Association,
Francis House,
Francis Street,
London SW1

Surfing

British Surfing Association,
56 Heol Glannant,
Ynysforgan,
Swansea

Swimming

Amateur Swimming
Association,
Harold Fern House,
Derby Square,
Loughborough,
Leics

National Association of
Swimming Clubs For the
Handicapped,
219 Preston Drove,
Brighton,
Sussex

Underwater swimming

British Sub-Aqua Club,
16 Upper Woburn Place,
London WC1

Water ski-ing

British Water Ski Federation,
16 Upper Woburn Place,
London WC1

Weightlifting

British Weight Lifters'
Association,
3 Iffley Turn,
Oxford

Windsurfing

Windsurfer Class Association
of GB,
c/o The Royal Yachting
Association,
Victoria Way,
Woking,
Surrey

Yoga

British Wheel of Yoga,
The Ramblers,
22 New Road,
Sandhurst,
Camberley,
Surrey

British Yoga Federation,
Aquarian House,
Clyn Ceiriog,
Llangollen,
Clwyd

SPORTS CENTRES/DANCE/ EXERCISE STUDIOS

Bodys,
250 King's Road,
London SW3

Dancercise,
Barge Durban,
Lion Wharf,
Old Isleworth,
Middlesex

The Hogarth Club,
1a Airedale Avenue,
Chiswick W4

Holmes Place Health Club,
Holmes Place,
188 Fulham Road,
London SW10

Pineapple Dance Centre,
7 Langley Street,
London WC2
and
60 Paddington Street,
London W1

Westside International Health
Centre,
201–207 Kensington High
Street,
London W8

YMCA,
HQ 640 Forest Road,
London E17
(write for your nearest sports
centre)

SPORTS EQUIPMENT SHOPS

Lillywhites Ltd,
Piccadilly Circus,
London SW1

Lonsdale Ltd,
21 Beak Street,
Regent Street,
London W1

Olympus Sports,
30 Oxford Street,
London WC1
(Branches in Manchester,
Leeds, Birmingham,
Liverpool, Bournemouth,
Ipswich, Colchester,
Peterborough)

The London Runner Shop,
Long Acre,
London WC2

Guide to chapter opening photographs

Chapter One/Page 11

I drive hundreds of miles each year in my SAAB Turbo 900. The seats are very comfortable, and I have adjusted them to accommodate my long legs. I think it is a good idea to stop in a lay-by for some stretching and neck exercises on a long drive.

Chapter Two/Page 19

I can use as many as twelve pairs of shoes in an event. Each pair is specifically designed for its job: warm-up shoes, javelin boots, discus shoes (wet weather), shot putt shoes, grass-running shoes, high jump shoes, 1500 m. shoes, discus (dry weather), long jump, 100 metres and 400 metres shoes, hurdles shoes, pole-vault shoes.

Chapter Three/Page 23

It is very important to maintain flexibility in your body and get rid of creaks before starting more strenuous exercises. Gillian, with me in the picture, is a busy mum who found my simple routine easy to do in her own sitting room.

Chapter Four/Page 31

This is the life! I did this daily exercise routine while learning to scuba-dive in the Cayman Islands, but life is not always quite so glamorous. With my Daley dozen, you can work out anywhere, at any time, whether you are on holiday in an exotic hotspot, or at home.

Chapter Five/Page 39

Even if you have only twenty minutes to spare each day, you can choose one of my workout routines and improve your shape. This exercise is one of the routines given in the *first* workout – for the fairly fit under-thirties in sedentary jobs. Not *me*, exactly, but perhaps you?

Chapter Six/Page 47

I use *any* method of transport to get to an athletics' meeting on time, including a private plane. This one is a bit more cramped than the jumbos our team usually travel in, but still adequate for isometric exercises. There is *no* space too confined for some kind of workout!

Chapter Seven/Page 51

Three's company, especially when we are a great team like this! My friends Gillian and Ryan (he is the adventurous two-year-old in the picture) really enjoyed the exercise session I organised in their home. How about joining us?

Chapter Eight/Page 59

Time: very early in the morning. *Place*: Battersea Park, London. *Temperature:* brrrrhh! Even on a chilly morning, running is fun if you are with friends like Helen and Snowy, and are dressed up really warmly. We had a lot of laughs and a good hot breakfast when we got home. A great way to start the day.

Chapter Nine/Page 67

Weight training covers a whole range of different exercise skills, from working out with dumb-bells, to doing a simple routine at home using a couple of baked bean tins. These kind of dumb-bells are preferable – easy to grip, and very professional looking.

Chapter Ten/Page 83

The 'Kids From Fame' had better watch out! Sylvia Caplin from London's Pineapple West Dance Studio put me through my paces in one of her classes. I enjoy dancing very much (and have been told I am quite good at it), so the routine we devised was tremendous fun.

Chapter Eleven/Page 91

Football is my second love after decathlon, and I play as often as possible. My young friends from the Coulsdon Colts FC in Surrey joined in these skills exercises. They were particularly good at the head tennis (page 99).

Chapter Twelve/Page 107

Swimming is fun, and superb exercise at any age. It is a vital part of any youngster's education to encourage him or her to develop confidence in the water. Sadly, not all schools have the resources for this, but local pools are usually reasonable, and grown-ups can benefit a great deal too.

Chapter Thirteen/Page 115

If you are going to stop for a snack, make sure it is a healthy one. I drink a *lot* of orange juice, and enjoy things like salad rolls, fruit and cheese when I get a break. Big Macs? I love 'em, but forget the French fries!

Chapter Fourteen/Page 123

This is the moment at the European Championships in Athens in August 1982 when all my planning *really* paid off! I had just crossed the line in the 1,500 metres, looked up at the board and found I had broken the world record. The picture won Steve Powell second place in the prestigious Adidas AIPs International Sports Photographer of the Year awards. (For technical fans: he used a Nikon F2 camera, 300 ml F28 lens, with Kodak EL 400 film, pushed 1½ stops, under floodlights, at 500th of a second at F28.)